Foreword by Dr. H.R. Nagendra, Chancellor, SVYASA University

YOGA VADE MECUM

Health Outcomes of Yoga Intervention

SUDHANVA CHAR

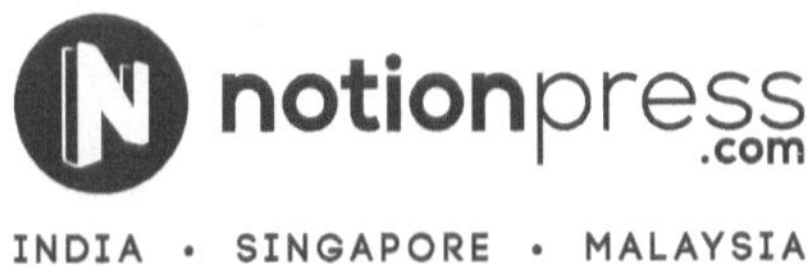

INDIA • SINGAPORE • MALAYSIA

Notion Press Media Pvt Ltd

No. 50, Chettiyar Agaram Main Road,
Vanagaram, Chennai, Tamil Nadu – 600 095

First Published by Notion Press 2021
Copyright © Sudhanva Char 2021
All Rights Reserved.

ISBN 978-1-63850-587-7

YUMMY YOGA NIBBLES

THE WELLNESS ASPIRATION THAT DEFINES YOGA LIFE STYLE

Pashyema Sharadashyatam | Jivema Sharadashyatam | Nandama Sharadashyatam |

*Modama Sharadashyatam | Bhavama Sharadashyatam
| Shrunuvama Sharadashyatam |*

Prabravama Sharadashyatam | Ajitasyama Sharadashyatam

Atharva Veda Hymn LXVII

Oh! Omniscient Sun-Lord, bless us so we may see for a hundred autumns, may we live for a hundred autumns, may we enjoy good life out of your abundance for a hundred autumns, may we imbibe deep (knowledge) for a hundred autumns, let us be and grow for a hundred autumns, let us listen to the scriptures well for a hundred autumns, may we bide and be invincible for a hundred autumns, may we thrive for a hundred autumns, and may we be so for even more than a hundred autumns!

Based on Hymns of the Atharva Veda by Ralph T.H. Griffith (1895), Sacred-Texts. Com

WELLNESS WISDOM

Sharira maadyam khalu dharma sadhanam

Sarga 5:33, Kumarasambhavam by Kalidasa

Only with a body in fine fettle any worthwhile goal can be attained.

Contents

Foreword to Yoga Vade Mecum

Dr. H.R. Nagendra M.E., Ph.D.
Chancellor, Swami Vivekananda Yoga Anusandhana Samsthana
(SVYASA University)
Bengaluru 560105, India

This book has the objective of presenting the reader with clinical and other evidence of the effectiveness of yoga intervention (YI) for some of the major health afflictions of mankind such as asthma, backache, cardiac concerns, cancer, COVID-19, depression and mental maladies, diabetes, genetic typos, geriatric issues of the elderly and other health problems. Throughout the book, anxiety and stress feature as the root causes of most of these challenges.

No one is under the illusion that yoga is a panacea for all health problems. However, together with ayurveda it guides people to robust physical and mental health that will stand any person in good stead in these times of a) hectic schedules, b) somewhat antagonistic environments, d) cognitive dissonance and d) more tempestuous forms of COVID-19.

At the end of the day, after one is done with the required yoga asanas, breathing exercises, kriyas, mudras and/or bandhas, one cannot but feel that yoga is more a discipline for being more mindful. It helps us take charge of our body, mind, emotions, and shunts aside life's absurdities and distractions in order to help us focus on life's goals. In this sense, yoga offers one of the best *modus operandi* to take charge of one's life and shape it in harmony with our values and principles.

Yoga Vade Mecum (YVM)

Compact handbooks are often called (in Latin) vade (go) mecum (with me). It is true there are hundreds of books on yoga and its different features and facets. So where is the need for another on yoga? This book is different. It tells about: a) the outcomes of scientific techniques of treatment and b) the clinical evidence there is of such benefits and side effects, and even adverse side effects, if at all any. This information would fill much needed gaps in evidence that seekers of yoga intervention as well as others in the health profession look for. But information becomes passé soon, thanks to the current dynamics of new research. It needs updating by endeavors like this compilation of new clinical evidence.

The yoga package consists of a) asanas b) *pranayama* and breathing exercises, c) mudras or subtle postures to deal with psychosomatic, emotive and prayerful intimations, d) cleansing exercises or kriyas such as dhouti, neti, nauli and others. The package includes e) bandhas such as jalandhara in the throat, uddiyana in the abdomen and moola in the perineum. The bandhas are for the purpose of locking prana in those parts of the anatomy and for asserting influence over those parts. There is meditation too in the package.

YVM would like to assist the reader locate solutions to health issues related to any critical body part or aspect of human physiology: the cardio-vascular, the digestive, endocrine, mental, reproductive, respiratory, excretive or musculo-skeletal systems. Yoga has a structured and systematic approach in this regard, and in regard to enigmas in life. This approach is spelled out in the across-the-board yoga methodology to any problematic state of affairs thanks to its evolution over millennia.

There are of course some who feel that yoga can hurt despite the evidence to the contrary. There are no side effects. Injuries can happen if students do not follow caveats, and do not heed cautionary signals. Study after study has determined that injuries seldom happen when students follow instructors and their advice. This topic has been covered in the YVM.

I thank the author for this persistent and spirited compilation which readers and health care professionals would find useful and even matter-of-fact.

H. R. Nagendra

Preface and Chapter Scheme

After a) an introductory review chapter of yoga, its ramifications, its competencies and proficiency in dealing with the major causes of death, and b) another chapter on the sizeable savings in health care costs without injuries and adverse side effects due to yoga intervention (YI), we should have gotten off to heart complaints as the number one cause of death as per the YVM original book-plan. The outcomes of yoga intervention (YI) were to be brought out according to the ranking in the Top Ten causes of death. However, an exception was made for COVID-19 in view of its topicality although it ranks third in causes of death. Number of deaths due to COVID-19 in India as of April 30, 2021 was nearly 212000. In the US, Coronavirus deaths were 526,483 as of March 05, 2021, as against 647,000 (2018) under heart-related and 606,520 (estimate for 2020) under cancer-related deaths. According to the National Safety Council over 47,600 Americans died of opioid-related overdose in 2017 – that's more than 130 lives each day. More recently, Health and Human Services reported that during the year ended June 2020 there were 83,000 drug overdose deaths in the USA. Morbidities of this kind too need to be addressed under psychological weak spots.

Second, besides providing effective therapy, yoga helps slash health care costs. In order to draw attention to this significant economic benefit of yoga modality, cost aspects too were brought in after COVID-19. The efficacy of breathing techniques for this SARS malady, together with the surprising cost-effectiveness of the modality would appeal to decision-makers.

Need for Larger Mandate for AYUSH

Whatever may be the persuasiveness of evidence from clinical trials, the fact is that yoga or ayurveda are not represented in health care decision-making anywhere in the world, not even in India, the home of yoga, except in an ad hoc way. There is of course the AYUSH (Ayurveda, Yoga, Unani, Siddha and Homeopathy) Ministry, Government of India, to take up the cause of those health modalities. While that may be so, practically all public health decisions are decided by professionals in conventional medicine who may or may not have expert knowledge about AYUSH modalities and their specialties. It is prudent that more integrated health care is expedited at least in India. That would enable ushering in an era of best practices, borrowing the best evidenced-based health care technique from any of the modalities. For this reason Chapter 4 was inserted to make a case for yoga, ayurveda and other AYUSH modalities in public health decision-making.

And still we were not ready to go for the heart. Yoga has an upper hand in resolving mental health problems and so we let Yoga and the Mind feature as Chapter 5 and Depression as Chapter 6. There are also related topics like Kundalini Chakra, GABA release, and migraine headaches. It then occurred that if we had already entertained COVID-19, how could we not drag in Yoga and the Immune System and the role of Lymph nodes? Not juxtaposing Coronavirus and the Immune system may be a faux pas. So Chapter 7 space got taken up by the human body's defense.

Chapter 8 has justified itself for yielding to Yoga and Common Sense, Cognition and Judgment. Its raison d'être is to bring home to readers that for sound health all that one needs to do are some basic Dos and DONTs: manage stress, belly breathe, avoid or minimize use of sugar, fat and carbs, watch your anthropometric measurements, don't smoke or drink, do yoga exercises methodically, do brisk walking, and such other common-sense steps which are otherwise critical for sound health. For instance, if the waist-hip ratio exceeds 1, there is higher risk of being overweight, and being vulnerable to heart disease and diabetes and/or cancer, more specifically for women. Breath or *prana* is a heavy-duty item in terms of criticality, but otherwise light as air. Hence the allocation of Chapter 8 to Common Sense in wellness.

Now it is time to bring in Heart? Wait a minute! Genes are the main reason offered for so many apparently healthy persons palpably in robust health, falling sick with cardiac, cancer, diabetes and other problems. Everyone knows of Indian Cricket Board President Sourav Ganguly, known to be hard-wearing and healthy, undergoing angioplasty twice in January 2021! That made us bring in Yoga and Genes up front in Chapter 9, and there is nothing impulsive about it!

Enough is enough, we said and brought in dear heart in Chapter 10. Cancer was waiting too long and got Chapter 11. Others to follow are Chapter 12 for Yoga Intervention (YI) in Asthma, Chapter 13 for YI in Diabetes (This deserves an earlier chapter rank, considering the legion of persons that is joining the diabetic fraternity with much higher risk of premature aging and death.) Chapter

14 is for YI for Back Pain. Who doesn't have backaches and neckaches? Hardly any exceptions other than the yoga folks!

Many pregnant women have learnt that the chances of reducing Caesarian section increases with yoga. The health of mother and the baby, (the future citizen!) improve too. So Chapter 15 was allotted to pregnancy. The topic of Chapter 16 is Yoga for Senior Citizens. The Chapter tells the elderly that people do not age uniformly, but at very different rates according to how much stress they have had in life and how much time they now give to yoga and fresh air.

And then comes the Epilogue: Yoga's role in keeping all Happy and Cheerful by tuning up the endocrine system, transforming our body into a smart biochemical factory. Annexure A is a recant of yoga philosophy and techniques. This is followed by Endnotes and Bibliography together.

Despite the name Yoga Vade Mecum, there are lacunae. For instance I could not include details of different asanas, mudras, breathing exercises, kriyas and bandhas by way of *materia medica* for remedial practices in yoga medicine. There are other shortfalls, such as not being able to be more comprehensive in offering clinical evidence or being more current. Another feature for which I seek your indulgence, is repetition of some basic facts about yoga, such as for example, parasympathetic nervous system domination rather than sympathetic nervous system, in different chapters. This was done to make each chapter somewhat self-contained, instead of making the reader go flipping back and forth to different pages in the book. Notwithstanding these drawbacks, I believe the current YVM serves a useful purpose, not just to yoga students and teachers, but to all other health care professionals engaged in ameliorating the human condition any which way! Friends that have read some chapters of YVM have opined that it would be desirable to have books like this as required texts in the area of complementary and alternative medicine so it may truly serve as a Vade Mecum.

Acknowledgements

YVM has been a few years in the making. At the annual yoga workshops in the Hindu Temple of Atlanta, Riverdale, GA since 1997 and at the Chinmaya Mission, Norcross, GA, as well as at corporate health workshops, and academic institutions, powerpoint presentations were made of new evidence of the outcomes of yoga intervention. My grateful thanks to HTA, CM, business firms, schools, colleges and charities for the opportunity to showcase yoga health benefits. So there was no need to start looking at health benefits of YI ab initio. Much of the evidence was there. They had to be consolidated and updated.

COVID-19 protocols confined me to Bengaluru, India and afforded me the time for updating and consolidating the evidence. However, for landing me this opportunity, no thanks to COVID-19, the mass slayer of innocent people and demolisher of economic, cultural and social progress.

I am grateful to Dr. H.R. Nagendra, with a monumental contribution to yoga research and education for his inspiring foreword. However, any errors of omission and commission in YVM are my own. I am also extremely thankful to wife Padma and family members for exempting me from family chores to work on the arduous tasks of research and compilation. Notion Press publication executives Anish Baskar and Pranav Wadhwa pressured me subtly to expedite this work. My thanks to them and their team.

List of Abbreviations

A-A	African-American
AA BCS	African American Breast Cancer Survivor
ACTH	Adrenocorticotropic Hormone
ADD	Attention Deficit Disorder
ADHD	Attention Deficit Hyperactivity Disorder
ADL	Activities of Daily Life
AHS	American Headache Society
AHA	American Heart Association
ATP	Adenine Triphosphate
ANOVA	Analysis of Variance
ANCOVA	Analysis of Covariance
ATGC	Adenine Thymine Guanine Cytosine order of bases in a segment of DNA molecules, the gene
AYUSH	Ayurveda Yoga Unani Siddha Homeopathy – Indigenous Alternative health modalities of India. Homeopathy is of German origin, but now indigenous enough. AYUSH Ministry oversees this health care system
BDI	Beck Depression Inventory
BP	Blood Pressure
BRCA 1 & 2	Breast Cancer Type 1 cell, Type 2 cell
CABG	Corona Artery Bypass Graft
CAD	Corona Artery Disease
CAM	Complementary and Alternative Medicine
CDCP	Centers for Disease Control and Prevention
CGI	Clinical Global Impression
CI	Confidence Interval for population parameters
COPD	Chronic Obstructive Pulmonary Disease
CPH	Cox's Proportional Hazards (model)
CRF	Corticosteroid Release Factor or Cancer Related Fatigue

CVD	Cardio Vascular Disease
COVID-19	Coronavirus Disease of 2019
DAL	Daily Activities of Life
DBP	Diastolic Blood Pressure
DHEA	Dehydroepiandrosterone
DMT2	Diabetes Mellitus Type 2
DNA	Deoxyribo Nucleic Acid
DSM-iv	Diagnostic and Statistical Mental Disorders Manual Forth Edition
EEG	Electroencephalograph
FDA	Food and Drug Administration
FSH	Follicle Stimulating Factor
GABA	Gamma Aminobutyric Acid
GDP	Gross Domestic Product
GDH	Gross Domestic Happiness
GH	Growth Hormone
GLM	Generalized Linear Model
GMO	Genetically Modified Organism
HDL	High Density Lipoprotein
HIV	Human Immunodeficiency Virus
HPA	Hypothalamus-Pituitary-Adrenal Axis
HPT	Hypertension
HRQoL	Health Related Quality of Life
HTA	Hindu Temple of Atlanta, Riverdale, GA
IDDM	Insulin Dependent Diabetes Mellitus (Type 1)
IDY	International Day of Yoga
IFN-γ	Interferon-gamma
IL-2R	Interleukin-2 Receptor
IOM	Institute of Medicine
KC	Kundalini Chakra
LDL	Low Density Lipoprotein
LSD	Lysergic Acid Diethylamide
LF/HF	Low frequency/high frequency
LH	Luteinizing Hormone
MAP	Mean Arterial Pressure
MBTT	Mind Body Transformation Therapy

MD	Mean Difference
MDD	Major Depressive Disorder
mtDNA	Mitochondrial DNA
NCHS	National Center for Health Statistics
NF-kB	Nuclear Factor kappa-light chain enhancer of B Cells
NIDDM	Non-insulin Dependent Diabetes Mellitus. Type II
NHIS	National Health Interview Survey
NIMH&NS	National Institute of Mental Health and Neuro Sciences
OHdG	8-hydroxy-2-deoxy-guanosine, a biomarker
OR	Odds Ratio
PBMC	Peripheral Blood Mononuclear Cell
PEFR	Peak Expiratory Flow Rate
PSA	Prostate Specific Antigen
PSNS	Parasympathetic Nervous System
PTSD	Post Traumatic Stress Disorder
QoL	Quality of Life
RDA	Recommended Dietary Allowance
RMANCOVA	Repeated Measures Analysis of Covariance
RNA	Ribonucleic Acid
RR	Relaxation Response. In Statistics, Relative Risk
RTC	Random Clinical Trials
SAU	Standard Arbitrary Units
SI	Suicide Ideation
SD	Standard Deviation
SDNN/ RMSSD	Standard Deviation of Normal to Normal (peak) point on graph/ Root Mean Square of Successive Differences
SMD	Standardized Mean Difference
SNS	Sympathetic Nervous System
SNOT	Sino Nasal Outcome Test
SBP	Systolic Blood Pressure
SARS	Severe Acute Respiratory Syndrome
STAI	State Trait Anxiety Inventory
TNF	Tumor Necrosis Factor
UI	Urinary Incontinence

WHO-QoL-BREF	World Health Organization Quality of Life Questionnaire Biomedical Reference (relating to physical, psychological, sociological and environmental factors.) Best Available Techniques Reference
WHO PANAS	WHO Positive and Negative Affect Schedule
HADS	WHO Hospital Anxiety and Depression Scale
YI	Yoga Intervention
YVM	Yoga Vade Mecum

Yoga's 'whatsoever' Faith

Under one of the limbs (*Niyamas* or Canons) of the 8-limb *(ashtanga)* yoga, for getting to anywhere in yoga, there is the tenet of a) *Iswara Pranidhana* or faith in God, along with four other tenets: b) *Shoucha* or mental and physical cleanliness c) *Santosha* or cheerfulness as a default state of mind d) *Swadhyaya* or learning all through life and e) *Tapa* or bringing to bear a stern outlook towards irrelevances in one's life. That's about it. Otherwise yoga is non-specific about one's spiritual faith. Any doubting Thomas, agnostic, theist or atheist can access and practice yoga for yoking and dovetailing of the amazing triad of mind, body and spirit, and can reap invaluable synergic benefits in life. Yoga philosophy has always been one of integrating all three dimensions into a single human persona, the parts working in perfect harmony, in step and style with each other. One cannot be good just in parts, but should be competent totally in all three dimensions to be able to perform best with all the cylinders firing in perfect sync.

Some faiths or institutions bar yoga practice. One example is the 1993 banning of yoga practice in Alabama schools by the State Board of Education because of its Hindu roots. By a March 2021 legislative action in the State House of Representatives and the State Senate, this ban is likely to be removed, but with the caveat that no original Sanskrit names of the exercises or other expressions such as Namasthe would be permitted. The reason for these conditions is the suspicion that yoga which is a spinoff of Hinduism, is a Trojan horse of that faith. This perception is rude to yoga as well as to the Hindu faith, because yoga is not that, and the faith does not care about proselytization! Yoga does not believe in converting anyone to anything other than rewarding robust health to any practioner.

Yoga, like the gracious faith itself, offers choice to the practioner. Like Georg Feuerstein would say, yoga is the consolidated wisdom of 200 generations, while all of American history is of 10 generations. Religious or other institutions barring someone from taking to yoga, deprive such a person of universal eternal wisdom for attaining energetic mind-body health and vital benefits therefrom.

Does learning allopathy as a modality of healing and fitness, together with the Hippocratic Oath, lead one to become a Christian? Does learning traditional Chinese mind and body exercises (TCMBE) like Tai Chi or Qigong make one a Chinese Marxist? Believing that yoga practice makes you a Hindu is that wacky! Who loses by banning people from taking to yoga? Surely, not Yoga: it has been making strides for eternity. The wellness loser is both the one who does not perform yoga as well as the community that decrees against its practice.

Yoga: Positives and Negatives

Positives

The text offers clinical evidence for the claims made below.

- Yoga is an anxiety and stress management champ. It helps brain cells generate Gamma Aminobutyric acid - GABA out of glutamate and daubs it on neurons in the brain to cut out chatter, and bring peace. GABA prohibits neuro-transmission or blocks bioelectric nerve impulses that may eventually fuse into thoughts. Thus, yoga is a bio-technique for sustaining *jiva* or the vital life force.
- Yoga invokes parasympathetic nervous system (PNS) and improves cardio-vascular efficacy. 'Fight or flight' resonation is moderated, absorbing the deleterious shock impact of more stress, instead of letting the sympathetic nervous system (SNS) get triggered by anxiety and stress.
- Slows aging and progression of arthritis, provides both alternative remedial and/or palliative cure for heart disease, diabetes, cancer, arthritis and osteoporosis. Strengthens musculo-skeletal system.
- Brings both remedial and prophylactic effects and serves as therapy for numerous ailments.
- Promotes objectivity, inner peace, positive feelings, self-confidence, stimulates initiatives to build society and promote welfare. It promotes natural joy.
- Ensures maximum functionality of body parts and mind, ensuring enduring physical and mental fitness and spiritual progress.
- Has proven credentials across eons. Over these ages there are no negative expositions/comments about yoga, other than the ones listed below!
- Practiced by millions worldwide (over 55 million in the US alone!) with appreciable wellness enhancements.
- Improves immunity against sickness invigorating the health of lymph nodes.

Negatives

- Devours some 30-40 minutes of precious time every day!
- Could cause injury when difficult asanas are done without teacher guidance.
- Criticized by some faiths to the extent of being barred from being practised by their followers. There is zero evidence of yoga not being secular or being exclusively religious with no choice. Yoga does not even ask the student to adhere to the Iswara Pranidhana tenet (Niyama). It is fine if out of one's own volition, the practioner absorbs tenets of Hindu faith like a) eschewing violence in thought, word and deed, b) being fearless under all circumstances, c) adhering to truth, appreciating one's dharma or life's rationale for presence on *terra firma*, d) thinking that actions or karma have consequences, e) bringing to bear moderation in emotions and consumption and f) being a wholesome human being.
- For the beginner there is a profligacy of yoga asanas, breathing, meditation methods, mudras, kriyas, bandhas, and practices. And then, there are terms in Sanskrit language: starting with the word yoga itself, (which otherwise has become part of the dictionary): *yama, niyama, asana, pranayama* and others mentioned in the last sentence. To make the situation more confounding, there are different yoga schools with no uniform coverage of any of the first four limbs of yoga: yama, niyama, asana and pranayama. Students, who later become distinguished teachers themselves, do not follow their own yoga teachers meticulously, and have fashioned their own distinctive 'gharanas' or schools of yoga! This is true of several celebrated teachers or gurus. For instance, some may teach just meditation and dub themselves yoga schools! May be there is nothing wrong in having blossoms of varied flowers in the yoga bouquet, but what happens to asana and pranayama and other limbs of yoga which should be there if it is yoga that is being imparted?
- To the person without a resolve (*sankalpa!*) to benefit from yoga, there is enough perplexity to agitate him or her to drop out! The uniform syllabus of the AYUSH Ministry (Government of India) could be an alternative to the uninitiated and others.[1] Yet another excellent reference book is Asana Pranayama Mudra Bandha by Swami Satyananda Saraswati, Yoga Publications Trust, Munger, Bihar, India. Beginners' classes can be simple, rigorous and effective enough to drive the aspirant to want to learn more and benefit more, health and wellness-wise.

Yogic Blessing: May robust yogic health make health insurance a huge surplus!

Yoga Vade Mecum - The Rationale

As the reader knows there are good many books on all aspects of yoga. However, for the lay person as well as the health professional, there are hardly any that tell about scientific if not clinical evidence as found in peer-reviewed journals and research papers. That is scientific validation of yoga. As the importance of yoga heightens, more and more people want to know of benefits and side effects of yoga bio-techniques, and even adverse side effects, if at all any. Further, research information becomes past its best quickly, necessitating updating. It should also refer to physical and mental conditions and complaints that yoga can take care of.

The array of yoga techniques include asanas, pranayama breathing exercises, mudras, cleanliness exercises or kriyas such as dhouti, neti, nauli, as well as bandhas and others. This is the yoga package of techniques with considerable heterogeneity, which is a plus factor for yoga applications, but somewhat of a negative feature when researchers do not identify or specify the practices in the yoga package that were imparted to the experimental group. This is essential if researchers want to replicate the clinical test and glean the same test outcomes. Evidence-based yoga would cite clinical trials with yoga interventions showing not just the success stories, but even the not so successful ones to minimize publication bias which however, cannot be avoided one hundred percent.

Yoga Vade Mecum (YVM) would like to assist the reader learn of solutions to health issues related to: the cardio-vascular, the digestive, endocrine, mental, reproductive, respiratory, or musculo-skeletal systems. Yoga evidence over these eternities panned out more like anecdotal evidence rather than in the form of clinical research and results thereof in articles in refereed journals like now, because there were none. Anecdotal evidence was also not questioned because of the integrity among yoga practioners and full trust in the gurus and vaidyas that deployed yoga or ayurveda techniques. There was little competition among the health care modalities. There were virtual best practices in India for treating health issues. The evidence, just for instance, was in the form of aphorisms and dicta, or Yoga Sutras of Patanjali, the expert affirmations in Swatmarama's Hatha

Yoga Pradipika, or the shat kriyas (six cleansing practices) for internal organs in Gheranda's Samhita, or Srinivasa Yogi's Hatha Ratnavali mentioning in detail the hows and whys of asanas and mudras. Today, in the midst of all scientific evidence, these sutras and dicta still remain invaluable reference. That reveals the cogency, precision and significance of the ancient texts such as Shiva Samhita urging all householders to practice yoga, and Yoga Vasishta underlining the primacy of the mind in wellness. 'Old is gold' is not an idle boast! However much exalted may be the integrity of past yoga annals, today's scientific research milieu demands validation in its very own style. Hence Yoga Vade Mecum!

Chapter 1

Yoga Vade Mecum

Yoga gets modish and spreads wings!

Yoga practice is spreading world-wide. But the same cannot be said about yoga philosophy and way of living. The latter are not put into practice to the same extent as the yoga drill. The uninitiated are willing to give yoga a try, but that is about it, nothing more. The author's 36-year long yoga teaching experience informs that they don't seem to have the longing for life style modification to avail of life improvements, as for example focusing on the goals of life, and eschewing life's irrelevances! That is tough and a tall order, not excluding for yoga practioners themsleves! But the fact is lifestyle diseases call for lifestyle changes! Changes of that kind seem to be far-fetched because much of yoga instruction anywhere in the world, is just for asanas together with some breathing exercises for the mind-body axis. Neither the American nor the Indian mind seems to have much of an appetite, leave alone craving, for the spiritual part of it or even the wellness part, as much as, for example, for pure hedonism, food and drinks, for ball games, cricket matches, music concerts, political developments, social get-togethers, hospital or clinic visits, electronic games and media like Face Book, Twitter, WhatsApp, TV and phones. Of course, this could be just an opinion, not revealed by hard evidence!

International Day of Yoga

Yoga finds home in over 150 countries, considering that out of 193 countries in the United Nations, 177 backed the International Yoga Day (IYD) UN Resolution sponsored by Prime Minister Narendra Modi in 2014 to launch the IYD effective June 21, 2015. IYD has given a stimulus to the global spread of yoga as a therapeutic way to address numerous health care issues besides fostering holistic mind-body fitness. Millions are evincing interest in yoga and learning it too, contributing to a beneficial impact on people's health, and their own and their country's health care bills. Even as the number of persons taking to yoga increases, so does the saving in health care costs. By resorting to yoga, there would be reduction in health care costs of about $500 billion in America alone as shown in Fig. 4. This estimate does not taking into account the conceivable savings arising from yogic exercises and breathing during the current COVID pandemic. Of course, the savings would materialize only if people take to yoga and become less vulnerable to the Coronavirus.

It should be puzzling that yoga, with so many benefits in terms of holistic wellness is still a far cry from being universally practiced in homes, schools, colleges, hospitals, workplaces and everywhere else. If yoga gains wider prevalence, America would go up several notches higher in wellness, and health care costs may plummet several levels down, depending upon how many people, patients and physicians opt for YI. Micro-decisions such as about breathing would have a macro benefit for American economy. In India the moot point is that if yoga had been a universal practice, the dimensions of the Coronavirus epidemic would have been far slighter. And so also the health care costs, the loss in production and economic activity, and even far less socioeconomic strife. There would be much less catastrophising of COVID-19 events. India, the land of yoga, should be able to highlight the gains, such as one of the lowest mortality rates (1.1% of infection cases as against world average of 2.2% in May 2021), even in the midst of the current second wave of COVID.

While yoga itself is becoming more widely known, it is far from becoming commonplace. There is of course, evidence of the spread. In America alone the number of persons practicing yoga techniques has gone up from 36.7 million in 2015 to 55 million in 2020.[2] This means just about 16.8% of Americans are into yoga. However, the increase of nearly 50% in 5 years cannot but be impressive. If this percent growth rate in the number of practioners is sustained, in 2025 their number would be around 70 million, about 20.1 percent of projected US population that year. If more people get more informed about the practice and its blessing of vigorous wellness there would be a groundswell of yoga adherents, a force for health. The percentage of population that needs to be vaccinated to attain herd immunity may be reduced if a large critical mass of a community, say 30% practice yoga.

Yoga has spread world-wide. In some countries the ancient practice has made much progress, described as staggering, like in Japan. There is not much statistics of yoga practice in Britain where it was introduced pretty early. Even if it is popular in terms of knowing about it, the growth of practioners appears to be tardy. Unlike in America, the number of practioners in Britain as a percent of the population is still in single digits, despite introduction there in the late 1800. It would be useful to have statistics about yoga conversant persons in different countries. One cannot avoid the misgiving that wherever medical health care is available on tap, there does not seem to be much of an incentive to seek yogic natural health. This is not very different from the complacency or the Peltzman effect spawned by safety belt, or air bags, or auto insurance in persons that tend to speed or drive rash. Similar smugness about one's health is imaginable if visits to clinics and hospitable are effortless and low-cost, or even gratis like under the world's largest health insurance cover fully funded by the Indian Government's Bharat Jan Arogya Yojana offering free insurance cover to 500 million Indians up to Rs. 500,000 per person.

Interesting information relevant to yoga usage was obtained from a cross-sectional survey of motivation for yoga, health benefits and behaviors in the UK.[3] This contrasts with an earlier survey in Table 7 about Medical conditions helped by Yoga presented on page 42. The data below is clearly indicative that yoga exercises are helpful, although the 'Helpful% ' goes down below 50% in the case of allergies and fertility issues, which are somewhat not well-defined medical terms otherwise.

Table 1: Perceived Percentage Helpfulness of Yoga in Managing Health Issues and Conditions

Condition	n*	Helpful%	Neither Helpful nor Unhelpful	Unhelpful%
Musculoskeletal				
Back Pain	1070	94.8	3.8	1.4
Neck Shoulder Pain	903	91.7	6.2	2.1
Arthritis	281	87.0	12.3	0.8
Other	424	82.8	2.4	
Mental Health				
Stress	997	98.4	1.4	0.2
Anxiety	712	96.8	2.9	0.2
Depression	513	93.2	5.5	1.4
Sleep Issues	463	79.0	19.7	1.2
Other	75	96.0	4	0
Women's Health				
Pre/Post Pregnancy	86	89.5	8.1	2.3
Pre-menopause Symptoms	275	76.5	22.5	0.7
Menopause	224	68.7	29.4	1.9
Other	98	77.6	21.4	1
Cardiovascular				
High Blood Pressure	160	73.0	26.3	0.6

Condition	n*	Helpful%	Neither Helpful nor Unhelpful	Unhelpful%
Other	57	66.7	31.6	1.8
Respiratory Issues				
Asthma	214	72.4	27.1	0.5
Other				
Gastrointestinal				
Irritable Bowel Syndrome	309	69.3	41.2	4.1
Other	96	68.4	22.3	2.7
Neurological				
Migraines	243	54.7	41.2	4.1
Headaches	475	68.7	22.3	22.7
Other	53	83.0	17	0
Other				
Allergies	296	27.2	66.4	6.4
Fertility Issues	74	32.4	58.1	9.5

*Number stating they had experienced the health condition/issue before/since practising yoga. Only conditions with responses >50 included.

Source: Cartwright T. et al. https://bmjopen.bmj.com/content/bmjopen/10/1/e031848.full.pdf

The main conclusion was that yoga practioners enjoyed higher health and well-being. They had lower risk behaviors as well as lower stress, BMI, and obesity. Initially they took to yoga because physical fitness was the objective. Over time however, the yoga choice was for psychospiritual factors. Yoga was also perceived as helpful for managing physical and psychological health issues. Yoga seemed to support self-care and manage health conditions. Also, over 90 percent of the yoga practioners were white, and have had college education.

Such granular data is not easily forthcoming for say India, Japan, USA, France, Germany and other countries. If analogous statistics were available for countries, it would help better decision-making about health matters, deriving sizable increases in wellness.

Emergence of Yoga Therapy or Yoga Chikitsa

There is little that is static in medical research. New findings crop up rapidly. It is not enough if scientific evidence of effectiveness of yoga therapy piles up. For its validation, the evidence needs to be organized disease-wise or medical complaint-wise like in Table 1 and then published in leading journals. Medical professionals have to be convinced enough to start prescribing yoga therapy. Medical schools do not teach alternative or complementary modalities and so this is hard. If nothing, yoga therapy professionals themselves have to be armed with gold standard scientific endorsement of their procedures.[4] This can then be deployed in utilitarian medical institutions besides yoga therapists themselves. At the least, organized evidence provides the first step to incorporate yoga practices like bellows and diaphragmatic breathing into the curriculums of medical schools. Second, it would also help yoga therapy get into the mainstream of health care instead of merely bob in its backwash. This has been the objective of annual Yoga Workshops at the Hindu Temple of Atlanta or the Chinmaya Mission, Norcross, GA.

Despite weaknesses in meta-analysis due to heterogeneity of exercises in the yoga package selected in RCTs by researchers, several of them have high methodological quality as well as control interventions in pain-associated disability and mental health.[5] This 2012 Summary of Reviews also entertained the view that yoga is a beneficial supportive/adjunctive treatment. It is relatively cost-effective. It provides life-long behavioral skills. It promotes self-confidence and has many other positive collateral benefits.

Today there is no dearth of clinical evidence of the effectiveness of yoga modality for a wide range of mental and physical problems. [6,7] There is increasing evidence that yoga ensures an equilibrium state of optimum wellness and health. Yoga is transforming, and can be deployed to up- or down-regulate phenotype, or the expression of a gene, but not (yet) the genotype or opening out of the actual genetic code. There has emerged "Medical Yoga Treatment (Yoga Chikitsa)" or the application of yoga techniques to ameliorate medical or health problems together with clinical evidence to support the claim that yoga is a fully-fledged therapeutic modality for many health issues. This is especially so for sickness that have origins in stress and tension.

Motives for doing yoga

The reasons given for taking to yoga in America are [8]

- Release tension (54%)
- Get stronger physically and mentally (52%)
- Feel happier (43%)
- Get more "me" time (27%)
- Feel less lonely (21%)
- Unplug from tech (20%)
  (Many respondents have ticked off more than one answer. That takes the total above 100%.)

Medical yoga intervention moves the patient towards wellness, both in terms of cure and prevention.[9] Yoga as a protocol increases the odds for longevity with vigorous health. It helps attain goals in life. Not long ago yoga was being hailed as "future medicine." That future appears nigh, just round the corner. It is worth underlining that YI is a behavioral intervention. To be successful, YI calls for active voluntary involvement of the participant rather than passive observation, at times with a cynic mind.

Anyone who practices yoga as regularly as he or she brushes teeth, will seldom fall sick or at the least, will get sick less often. Despite regular exercise and precautions, should sickness come about due to infections and/or pollution of food, water or air, the body's immune mechanism kicks in adeptly, homeostasis sets in and the body is restored to normal health relatively quickly. For instance, a person who practices yoga may recover from a cold or fever after say twelve hours of rest; whereas other persons may take a few days. Isn't that a big difference? (See Opinion Survey of Yoga practioners on page 31) When travelling, it is all the more important that we set aside time for yoga because it will help the body and mind to calibrate themselves to the new (circadian) environment at the destination.

Holistic Outlook and Taming Stress

Yoga has much appeal as a health modality because it is not piecemeal, fixated on just the symptoms. There are no side effects of yoga treatment done per instructions. Like ayurveda, yoga therapy believes that one size does not fit all, and therefore any treatment has to be individualized according to the physiological and psychological makeup of the patient.

Yoga practice for fitness can however, be common to all and even here, some personalization may call for different *stresses* on *sukshma* (or subtle) asanas and *sthoola* (heavy duty) *vyayama* or exercises, as well as selections from mudras, breathing exercises, kriyas, and bandhas, which we call the yoga package. Yoga goes much beyond just the symptoms. It tackles the root causes of any given health problem. And so the remedy is not fractional like in some modalities, but its solutions are more cohesive, global and all-inclusive. It is personalized like Ayurveda medication. Ayurveda treatment is based on individual *vata, pitha and kaffa doshas* and other distinctions between people, including genes, genders and life styles. Primary proficiency of yoga treatment lies in its uncanny ability to tame the beast of stress. Stress kick-starts Hans Selye's 'fight or flight' nerve reaction. Medical Hall of Fame endocrinologist Selye came up with the General Adaptation Syndrome to theorize that if people to do not learn to cope with the stressors, they will have adverse health outcomes such as ulcers, high blood pressure, and even heart attacks. There are five stages of stress: alarm, resistance, possible recovery, adaptation and burnout.

Not Activating H-P-A Axis and Not Generating Cortisol

The yoga practioner, however, is able to cope with stressors according to one's stress-tolerance capability and stay cool even if the tiger of stress is posing a visible threat. Yoga ensures that the practioner is unflappable and stays calm. It does this, with not just GABA, but also by invoking the parasympathetic nervous system (PSN) rather than habitually resorting to the sympathetic nervous system (SNS). When we are assaulted constantly by a volley of anxieties and stresses the SNS is at its wit's end and soon there is burnout. On the other hand, the PSN is like a shock-absorber for stress, absorbing all the anxiety and panic attacks. And yet it may not activate very much the neuroendocrine arrangement called the hypothalamus-pituitary-adrenal (HPA) axis, in the process not generating as much corticosteroid as the SNS. Stress and fear produce vasopressin and corticotrophin-release- hormones (CRH) in the hypothalamus. The two biochemicals in turn stimulate generation of adrenocorticotrophic hormone (ACTH) in the pituitary. ACTH goes on to stimulate cortisol in the adrenal glands. These processes have both salutary and adverse impact on homeostasis, the immune system, metabolism, cardiovascular system, reproduction and of course, the central nervous system. Such a chain reaction in a sequence could operate like the domino effect and increase vulnerability to diabetes, insomnia, irritability, infections, bone fractures and others. There are also fatigue and burnout. The quality of life goes down, and the end could not be far away.

The Telomerase Enzyme

It is now corroborated that stress shortens life spans and one bit of evidence lies, *inter alia*, in telomeres at each end of chromosomes. Chromosomes carry the genetic code or the genes, and reside in the nucleus of human body cells. They are basically repetitive nucleotide sequences. *Telos* in Greek means end and *meros* means part. Telomeres, sustained by the telomerase enzyme, prevent damage to chromosomes and extend the life span of cells. Their length correlates with stress, shorter telomeres with more stress and vice versa. Yoga, meditation and other mind-body training, protect and maintain the length of telomeres. If this is so, it serves as scientific validation of yoga's impact on longevity at the gene/genome level. [10,11] The Ornish pilot study (2013) looked into the possible transformation of telomerase activity and associated telomere maintenance capacity in human immune-system cells. Cellular enzyme telomerase counteracts telomere shortening. The lifestyle factors that nurture cancer and cardiovascular disease also impact telomerase function. Yoga practices such as asanas, pranayama and meditation prevent oxidative DNA damage and cellular aging. They protect the ends of telomeres and ensure genomic integrity.

Telomere Length as Prognostic Marker

The Ornish pilot study recruited 30 men with biopsy diagnosed low-risk prostate cancer and asked them to go for comprehensive lifestyle changes, examples of which would include nutrition, yogic exercise and breathing, sound sleep, stress-free social and work ecosystem, right music, clean air and clean water consumption. The investigators were tracking telomerase enzymatic activity per viable cell measured both at baseline and after 3 months of intensive lifestyle and nutrition improvements.

The research question the study wanted to answer was whether improvements in nutrition and lifestyle would also improve telomerase activity in peripheral blood mononuclear cells or PBMC. The results were that PBMC telomerase activity expressed as natural logarithms ($\log_e$) increased from 2.00 (Standard Deviation 0.44) to 2.22 (SD 0.49; p = 0.031). Raw values of telomerase increased from 8.05 (SD 3.50) standard arbitrary units (SAU) to 10.38 (SD 6.01) SAU. There was significant association between increases in telomerase activity and decreases in low-density lipoprotein (LDL) cholesterol (**r**=−0·36, p=0·041) and also decreases in psychological distress (**r**=−0·35, p=0·047). The study concluded that comprehensive lifestyle changes, including yoga exercises, significantly increase telomerase activity and which in turn impact telomere maintenance capacity in human immune-system cells. The study was rightly shy of terming the significant association between these variables as a causal factor without more random controlled trials. However, changes in telomere lengths in human beings is emerging as a prognostic marker of disease risk, progression, and premature mortality in many types of cancer, including breast, prostate, colorectal, bladder, head and neck, lung, and renal cell.

The Immortality Enzyme

There is new evidence that yoga-based life-style intervention would help reduce levels of oxidative stress and cellular aging in obese men. One particular 2015 research work[12] at the All India Institute of Medical Sciences, New Delhi is a case study of a 31-year old person with class I obesity (BMI 29.5 kg/m$_2$)

who complained of extreme fatigue, problems in losing weight, and lack of motivation. The objective was to assess the impact of yoga intervention on levels of biochemical markers such as cellular ageing, oxidative stress and inflammation at three time lines: baseline (day 0), end of active intervention (day 10) and follow up on day 90. The person also stated that there was a marked decrease in energy level in the afternoons. He was introduced to asanas, pranayama, stress management, group discussions, lectures and individualized advice. The results were, as shown in Table 2, significant increases in a) telomerase in the period from day 0 to day 10 and again to the follow up day 90, b) the activity of telomerase and c) levels of β-endorphin. In the same period d) plasma cortisol and interleukin-6 decreased, and e) there was a sustained reduction in oxidative stress markers, such as reactive oxygen species (ROS) and 8-hydroxy-2-deoxy-guanosine (OHdG) levels. Yoga helps reverse markers of aging such as oxidative stress, telomerase activity and oxidative DNA damage. There are hints that youthful healthy life can be induced to serve as therapy for such damage, encouraging the naming of telomerase as the immortality enzyme.

Table 2: Yoga and Telomerase Enzyme

Variable	Baseline (Day 0)	End of Active Intervention (Day 10)	FollowUp (Day 90)
Telomerase(IU/Cell)	0.72	2.80	37.4
ROS (RLU/Min per 10^4 neutrophils)	1422.069	1190.81	1005.01
8-OHdG (pg/mL)	11,205.75	9863.11	6467.32
Cortisol (ng/mL)	121.08	98.12	93.30
Interleukin-6 (pg/mL)	2.73	2.11	1.90
β-endorphin (pg/mL)	3.53	4.06	6.313
8-OHdG, 8-hydroxy 2'deoxyguanosine; RLU - relative light unit; ROS - reactive oxygen species			

Source: Kumar SB et al 2015

DNA and the Environment

Dynamic DNA (2018) by Sharma et al mentions an earlier study of Sharma et al (2008) which evidences the influence of the living environment on DNA. The influence of the ecosystem cannot be underestimated. This is because the DNA is watching the host person 24/7 and sees, listens, thinks everything the person sees, listens and thinks. So if the host is listening to mellow music, the resident DNA is also doing the same and thinking the same. This applies to both good deeds and bad, and their impact on DNA. Whatever our ancestors did, it is in our DNA and will be there in our grandkids' DNA unless such an inherited baggage of lineages is jettisoned and transformed through right listening, right speaking, right thinking and so forth. In a way, this DNA lesson is inherent and embodied in all. We will look into phenotype and genotype too, a little later under Yoga and Genes.

Yoga's Deep Connection

Yatha Brahmande, tatha pindande – As is the universe or the macrocosm, so is the microcosm. This ancient wisdom is now adumbrated in science. It goes like this: The brain consists of 100 billion neurons with trillions of connections. Astrophysicists and neuroscientists are now agreeing that the complexity of the universe is similar to that of the brain, including their structures. "The universe may be self-similar across scales that differ in size by a fraction of a billion billion billion."[13] (yes, the word billion repeats itself 3 times, not an error!) *Brahmanda* is the initial egg of creation of the universe and *Pindanda* is the cell-level or embryonic egg. Ayurveda and yoga relate themselves to this through the 25 elements including the five mahabhutas of air, water, earth, ether and fire, as per Sankya philosophy and consider the human body a hologram of the universe. What is not in the body is not anywhere else, in particular the 118 elements in the Periodic Table of Chemical Elements such as hydrogen, oxygen, sodium, carbon, helium, chlorine, lithium, iron, gold, lead, calcium, copper, nitrogen, sulphur, magnesium and so forth. This perception of connections to the origin is fully recognized in the ancient system of medicine. It is in the light of this profound perception that treatment is fine-tuned. The manifest objects are ever-changing like the world, but the unmanifest never-changing aspects with deep connections to the universe are embedded perhaps in the genes. YA (yoga-ayurveda) go this deep to the genes themselves to heal, if need be.

For treatment success it helps if people with medical complaints do not wait long before trying out YA. YA should have the first shot at cancer, most cardiovascular and other complaints. In practice, YA is indeed the last resort after some stay at the hospice. Thus there is the case of 34-year old Amit Vaidya, badgered by cancer during his life in America and then miraculously made cancer free by *panchagavya* and cow dung and so forth.[14,15] In 2012 Vaidya's oncologist in the US told him that his cancer had spread from the stomach to the lungs, liver and spine in spite of countless chemo sessions, radiation and two clinical trials. The prognosis was that he had six months to live. He was exhausted with chemotherapy and radiation right up to the frustration point. He decided to return to India to breathe his last there. On the spur of someone's suggestion, he stoically agreed to try Ayurvedic *Panchgavya* treatment in a hospital in Gujarat. Many like him appear to win the cancer battles, but are really losing the cancer war. But panchagavya saved him from cancer. He salvaged himself from his "chemo brain" and its disdainful thoughts. He was cancer-free. All this for an astoundingly non-price of one rupee (yes, one rupee for the lifesaving treatment and 11 day stay in the hospital, and the diet.) Now Amit Vaidya lives hale and hearty on the backwaters of Kerala many years beyond his literal deadline.

YA should not be the last resort after using up all energies and resources in treatments such as chemotherapy and radiation as in the case of cancer, or steroids and other medications. There could be Pyrrhic victories gaining tactical advantages over cancer cells, but eventually losing life to cancer. Yoga, with its universal and global perspective, makes a dysfunctional part functional when enabled as such. Old life styles and old samskaras or net results of one's positive and negative karmas or activities may still be there in the neural networks. And yet lifestyle change can occur with sankalpa. This is the ability of the brain to build new synoptic connections particularly after some reeducation or injury, as it happens in neuroplasticity which at any age can create its own neural pathways. Daily yoga practice is a great prophylactic as well as a cure for several health problems demanding new synoptic pathways.

Can Yoga be Secular?

While the world may hail almost in a consensus that yoga promotes all round mental and physical fitness, besides making overtures to the spiritual dimension, for the sake of persons rooted in different faiths, yoga is characterized also as a secular activity. One does not feel any obligation to chant Hindu words like *Namaste, Om* or *Jai* or *Vande Gurum* etc. Yoga instruction anywhere is catholic enough to let people articulate whatever they wish to either before, during or after the yoga asanas, breathing, meditation and any other protocol. A British psychiatrist says: "Although yoga has its origins in Indian religion, it can be practised secularly and has been used clinically as a therapeutic intervention."[16] Not surprisingly therefore some 14 million persons have been recommended by their physicians to take to yoga for numerous problems.[17]

By mischaracterizing it as a Hindu religious activity, many believers of other faiths have been led to sidestep yoga. The 1993 Alabama Board of Education decision banning yoga in schools has been mentioned earlier. This is sad because first it is not a religious activity. Second, yoga is not a Trojan horse to introduce any religion. Third, the misrepresentation is costing the believers of those faiths much wisdom for fostering physical and mental health at virtually no cost, keeping the health care costs down and otherwise enjoying full-bodied health in all weathers, fair or foul, without any special exercise gear other than whatever people are wearing and in the comfort of one's home. Not once in the last 30 years or so that Americans including African-Americans have been attending yoga classes in the Hindu Temple of Atlanta, Riverdale, GA they have been told to embrace any particular faith. Thoughts like converting people of other faiths don't even flash on our mind. There is laser focus on just imparting yoga knowledge.

Anxiety-ridden World

Yoga is obsessed with wellness and longevity, so apparent from the Atharva Veda quote under 'Yummy Yoga Nibbles' on the opening page v. The collective gain to society from a majority of the nation's population whether in India or in America or in the world practicing yoga and enjoying all-round fitness would be stunning. The Gross National Product (GDP) would achieve its potential with all the factors of production, 'labor' in particular, at full play, and so would the Gross National Wellness and Happiness! Let us call it GDH. Incidentally America ranks number one in GDP, but ranks 18th in happiness in a world-wide United Nations ranking of 156 countries.[18]

One can imagine the overwhelming issues that confronts densely-populated countries like India which figure at the bottom of the World Happiness scores. The scores are composite totals of numerical credits derived from measures like per capita Gross Domestic Product, Healthy Life Expectation at birth, social support, freedom to make life choices, generosity in terms of donations made, corruption perception, and related factors. America's rank is 18 with a score of 6.940 against number one Finland's 7.809. Most Nordic countries are 7 and above. Currently India's score is 3.573, and disappointingly, ranks below Bangladesh, Myanmar, Haiti and Sri Lanka and is only ahead of Afghanistan's score of 2.567.

If India pushes forward with yoga for the masses, in particular the rearward sections of society like the Dalits or Harijans, India's rank would leap ahead of a hundred countries. This would happen in view of the substantial contribution that yoga would make to productivity and per capita GDP, life expectation by boosting health at virtually insignificant cost, improving fellow feeling and harmony, freedom to make better decisions and choices for better quality of life, more ethical liberal living and less corruption, simple living and high thinking, and so forth.

GDP-GDH Gap

Needless to say that the gap between the two per capita measurements of Product and Happiness is too wide for America, and much worse for India! This predicament guides how we need to make America, India and/or the world great! And as a matter of fact India was Numero Uno in its GDP size (and possibly in per capita too) compared to any other nation in the world till 1600 AD, accounting for almost a third of world GDP. After that there was colonialism and exploitation reducing India's GDP. And yet, it ranked at the very top, second only to China till 1700. [19.] Thereafter there was the proverbial Gadarene descent for both India and China. India has a long way to go in getting back to higher ranks in GDP and GDH. Universal practice of yoga can help India get back there fast. It is difficult to tell anything about GDH in China despite the obvious higher material standards.

No one should translate these thoughts as an audacious claim that yoga is a magic or silver bullet for all problems. That is not even implied. What is without a doubt true, and well-substantiated by evidence on the pages to follow, is that if life style changes are assimilated, yogic and ayurvedic ways of life are adopted, there is an excellent prospect of a great boost in productivity following good health and wellness of people. This could be leveraged for augmenting progress and development in other walks of life and in nation-building. Nothing more or nothing less is suggested about yoga, certainly not a universal remedy.

Yoga is without doubt, not a flash in the pan. It has been examined thoroughly by world's rational and discerning public and medical professionals for a few millennia. In recent years it has helped many hundreds of thousands overcome the trammels of sickness and enjoy full-bodied health. Yoga is also unique in creating the environment that serves as a disinfectant and decontaminator vis-à-vis physical and mental diseases and even genetic disorders, not to speak of holistic peace with oneself, and being at peace with the outside world.

Take for example the research papers in just English language medical journals such as Lancet, JAMA *(Journal of the American Medical Association)* or *NEJM (New England Journal of Medicine)* over the past sixty years or more, and note the wide range of physical and mental ailments that "medical yoga" is legitimately credited as holding out hope for either as a prophylactic or even a cure.[20] The references relate to application of yoga therapy for disparate ailments and conditions: addictions like smoking, drinking alcohol-based beverages, hallucinogens, sickness like asthma, Alzheimer's, anxiety disorder, backache, breathing issues, depression, diabetes, dyspnea, menopause, post-menopausal osteoporosis, fibromyalgia, cancer, health coaching, heart diseases and hypertension, reactions to LSD, carpal tunnel syndrome, mental health, sciatica, stress management, visceral functions, relaxation response, angina pectoris, bio-behavioral approach to pain, evolution of human behavior, and so forth. This should clear doubts about the range of health problems that the principles of yoga modality are being applied to.

Yoga rests its case for total health in all three dimensions as an essential component of its holistic philosophy, its strong suit. Equally, if not more critically, medical yoga's uniqueness lies in putting into play the parasympathetic nervous system (PSNS) to handle stress routinely. Yoga spares the already overloaded and abused sympathetic nervous system (SNS) from managing stress. When SNS goes on overdrive with a sustained activation of the hypothalamus-pituitary-adrenal (HPA) axis, as already stated on page 7, there is excessive release of corticosteroid, a hormone produced in the cortex of the adrenal glands. It has the advantage of reducing inflammation and preparing for 'fight or flight' situations. But over a longer period, it may increase blood sugar, cause insomnia, increase irritability, bring mood changes, affect bone density increasing vulnerability for fracture, and also make one susceptible for infections by suppressing the immune system. If this set of circumstances comes about, the immune system may attack its own tissues mistaking them as foreign.

Yoga Usage

According to a 2017 National Health Interview Survey (NHIS) the use of yoga, meditation and chiropractic went up during 2012-17.[21] The Report was brought out by both the National Center for Complementary and Integrative Health as well as the National Center for Health Statistics (NCHS) of the US Centers for Disease Control and Prevention (CDCP). Every five years a questionnaire is administered and many thousands of Americans are interviewed about their health and illness. The findings are published as NCHS Data Brief. The highlights of this latest report are tabulated below and the following demographic data are also given:

- Use of yoga, meditation, and chiropractic among Non-Hispanic white adults was more likely compared with Hispanic and non-Hispanic black adults.
- Adults aged 18 to 44 years compared to older adults, used yoga the most, while the use of meditation and chiropractic care was higher among adults aged 45 to 64 years compared with younger and older age groups.

Table 3: Yoga-Meditation Demographics - Percentage of Adults using Yoga, Meditation and Chiropractic

Percentage Increases	2012	2017
Yoga	9.5	14.3
Meditation	4.1	14.2
Chiropractic	9.1	10.3
Gender wise use	**Men**	**Women**
Yoga	8.6	19.8
Meditation	11.8	16.3
Chiropractic	9.4	11.1

Source: NCHS Data Brief

Yoga Injuries

As yoga practioners can vouch, the probability of injuries is very low in the course of doing yoga under a certified yoga instructor. This does not mean that there can be no injuries at all. There may be persons overenthusiastic about learning the more difficult asanas such as for instance *dwipada shirasana* (or two feet to head) pose or *Vrischikasana* (the scorpion pose). No teacher worth the salt would not tell in advance the contra-indications of each asana or pose, or even pranayama or abdominal breathing. The data given below in Fig.1 and Fig.2 do not give the information regarding:

a) Which asanas the injured person tried and suffered a sprain or got into some trouble.
b) Was he/she doing the exercise under guidance or on his/her own?
c) Was the person aware of the contraindications?
d) Was the person a beginner or an advanced yoga practioner?
e) Was the person in a hurry of some kind to complete the asana and not mindful enough?

Another important lesson for avoiding injuries is to have an instructor like BKS Iyengar, known to be harsh in class, offering only tough love, and yet who understood a student's personal needs and taught the yoga asanas according to the student's special requirements. He learnt from his own teacher Krishnamachar that injuries happen because students strain themselves in difficult poses. If helped with props such injuries may not happen, and gradually as the student learns, one can give them up. Props included sand bags, bricks, towels, things rolled inside blankets, strings/slings latched on to walls, and others. Props helped students to relax into a pose and destress themselves even as their breath improved.[22] The tension is gone and natural balances are restored. A feeling of safety is enjoyed while doing individualized yoga.

Take the case of not following the safety procedures and safeguards. Let us say someone is attempting shirshasana or headstand. When a person is doing it for the first time it is important that the instructor is present and preferably the learner does the exercise against a wall. While doing it the probability of losing balance and falling off on the back side is very high. Instructors compel beginners to do it against the wall, preferably a corner in the room, with some minimum cushioning for the head with a carpet or a rug or a yoga mat. Doing in a corner ensures support from three sides in the case of a fall. Many beginners try doing the headstand without wall or pillar support and without adequate cushion buttress for the head. Such noncompliance cannot but end up in some neck or back injury. Secondly, from personal experience, this author can say that minor sprains and other injuries have occurred when children are around. Clowning around, grandkids have pushed me off balance, but luckily no injury was there.

Imitating the Leaning Tower of Pisa

When visiting the Leaning Tower of Pisa in 2018, I imitated it by curving my torso and legs to a side while doing shirshasana on grass with a hand kerchief under my head. The grass under was cushion enough. I was in a hurry to complete the pose so I could catch up with the family that was moving away from the tourist spot. Nevertheless, I was able to complete the imitation of the Tower in the headstand pose and no injury happened. But this is an illustration of how not to rush and ignore safety. On an earlier occasion, decades ago a naughty child picked up an expensive watch I was keeping in front of my face to time my headstand, and threw it off the 5th floor balcony. I had to get off my pose in a hurry and could not complete the 3-minute shavasana one is required to do after a head stand. As a result it is possible that the positive effects of the headstand and shavasana got commuted.

All instructions need to be scrupulously followed and instructors need to enforce them for their own business solvency to prevent claims happening from injured yoga students. This is one of the reasons for the increase in number of yoga instructors buying malpractice insurance. Fortunately, as statistics show in Fig 1 and Fig 2, the number of injuries per 100,000 is still in single digits, unless different injuries to head, lower limb, trunk and other parts are added up such as 17 injuries in 2014 (Fig. 2: 3.49 + 3.92 + 0.50 + 8.41 + 0.69). The injury numbers are not even comparable to those in many sports: football, soccer, or basketball. The conspicuous turns and twists in the curves relate to persons 65 years and older in the first graph and injuries to the trunk in the second graph.

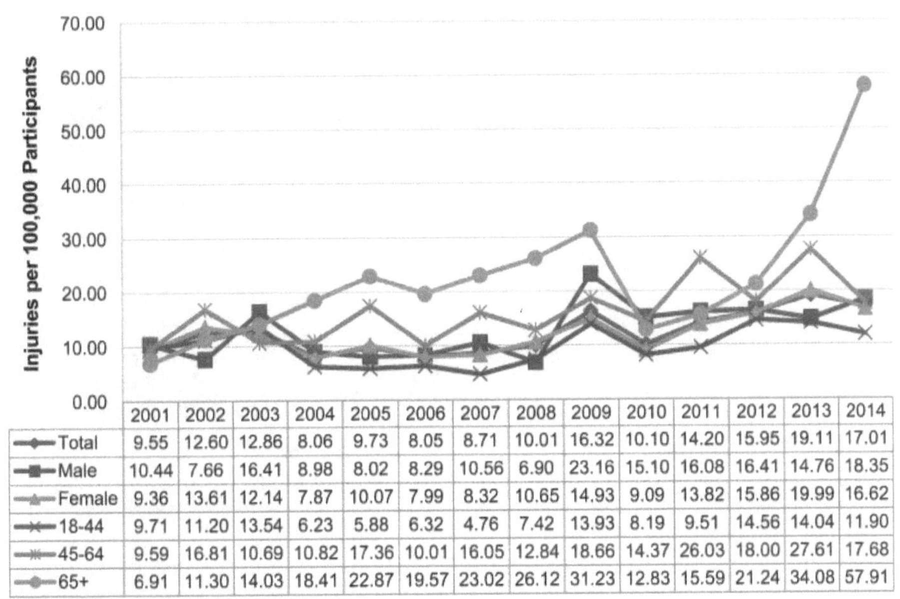

	2001	2002	2003	2004	2005	2006	2007	2008	2009	2010	2011	2012	2013	2014
Total	9.55	12.60	12.86	8.06	9.73	8.05	8.71	10.01	16.32	10.10	14.20	15.95	19.11	17.01
Male	10.44	7.66	16.41	8.98	8.02	8.29	10.56	6.90	23.16	15.10	16.08	16.41	14.76	18.35
Female	9.36	13.61	12.14	7.87	10.07	7.99	8.32	10.65	14.93	9.09	13.82	15.86	19.99	16.62
18-44	9.71	11.20	13.54	6.23	5.88	6.32	4.76	7.42	13.93	8.19	9.51	14.56	14.04	11.90
45-64	9.59	16.81	10.69	10.82	17.36	10.01	16.05	12.84	18.66	14.37	26.03	18.00	27.61	17.68
65+	6.91	11.30	14.03	18.41	22.87	19.57	23.02	26.12	31.23	12.83	15.59	21.24	34.08	57.91

Graph 1. Injuries by Age Groups

Source: Swain TA, McGwin G. Yoga-Related Injuries in the United States From 2001 to 2014. Orthop J Sports Med. 2016 Nov 16;4(11):2325967116671703. doi: 10.1177/2325967116671703. PMID: 27896293; PMCID: PMC5117171.

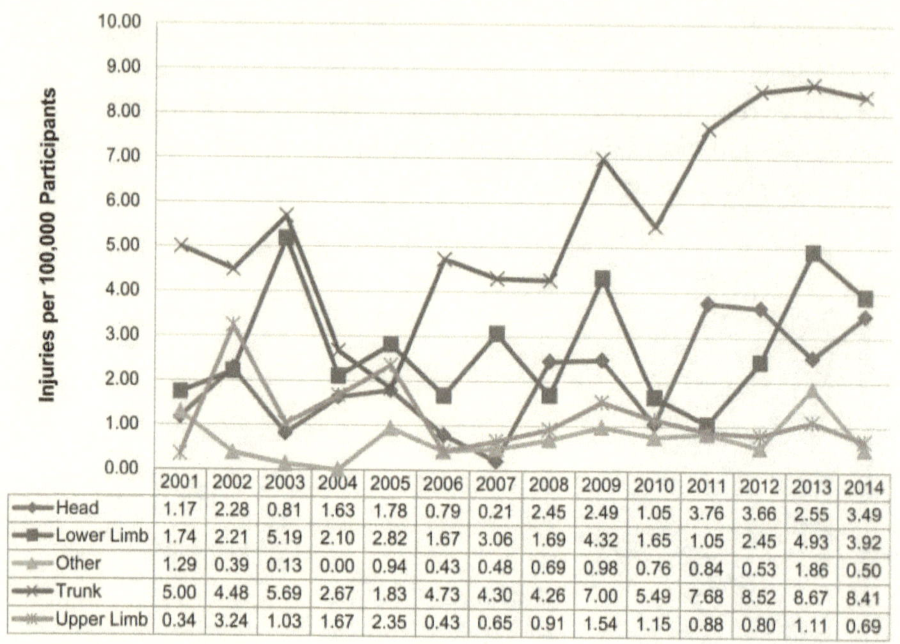

	2001	2002	2003	2004	2005	2006	2007	2008	2009	2010	2011	2012	2013	2014
Head	1.17	2.28	0.81	1.63	1.78	0.79	0.21	2.45	2.49	1.05	3.76	3.66	2.55	3.49
Lower Limb	1.74	2.21	5.19	2.10	2.82	1.67	3.06	1.69	4.32	1.65	1.05	2.45	4.93	3.92
Other	1.29	0.39	0.13	0.00	0.94	0.43	0.48	0.69	0.98	0.76	0.84	0.53	1.86	0.50
Trunk	5.00	4.48	5.69	2.67	1.83	4.73	4.30	4.26	7.00	5.49	7.68	8.52	8.67	8.41
Upper Limb	0.34	3.24	1.03	1.67	2.35	0.43	0.65	0.91	1.54	1.15	0.88	0.80	1.11	0.69

Graph 2. Injuries by Body Parts

Source: Swain et al Ibid

There are no fatal injuries in yoga. Individuals with preconditions need to perform exercises, even simple exercises such as pranayama under supervision. The age of a majority of persons that got injured was 65 years or more. Beginners as a rule should start with some of the simplest of exercises not involving lumbar twists, and avoid alcoholic beverages especially before exercises. A 2013 study found that 35.5% of the total incidents affected the musculoskeletal system, 18.4% the nervous system and 11.8% the eyes.[23] With the exception of one or two incidents, most of them were temporary injuries and got cured in quick time. Thus injuries are not even an issue when caution and mindfulness are put into effect while performing the exercises.

Motivations for Yoga

According to a 2012 survey 94 percent of adults practiced yoga for wellness reasons and 17.5 percent to address a specific health condition. (The totals add up to more than 100 because some opted for both the reasons.) [24] What was interesting in the Survey was what the adults said about how yoga helped them:

• 86 percent said it reduced stress

- 67 percent said it helped them feel better emotionally
- 63 percent said it motivated them to exercise more regularly
- 59 percent said it improved sleep
- 82 percent said it improved overall health and made them feel better.

Other reasons were also given for taking to yoga

- 43 percent said yoga motivated them to eat healthier
- 39 percent said yoga helped coping with health problems
- 25 percent of people who currently smoke cigarettes said yoga motivated them to cut back or stop smoking cigarettes
- 12 percent of people who currently drink alcohol said yoga motivated them to cut back or stop drinking alcohol.

There do not appear to be many differences when the motives listed above are contrasted with those listed on page 5 above. But those motives for taking to yoga appear to be different for age groups. Middle-age groups believed it would help increase muscle strength and help lose weight. Older adults were interested in yoga to mitigate or eliminate health issues related to age. A survey of veterans showed that women were more interested in yoga than men for their backache.

Some Anecdotal Instances

One of the objectives of YVM, as noted above, is the offering of clinical evidence of effectiveness of yoga intervention in health issues. There is much clinical as well as anecdotal evidence to make decisions about yoga intervention in the treatment of various illness and adverse health conditions. Before getting down to clinical trials, it would be interesting to learn what anecdotal evidences have to reveal, giving them brownie points for any useful information. Case studies at times spill beans ahead of clinical research and help researchers to warm up to clinical trials! Anecdotal evidence, for instance tells that interest in yoga exercise is often as a result of not receiving adequate resolution of an existing health problem through other modalities. The thought process is: "Well, I have tried medication, surgery and other treatments. There is no change in my morbidity status. So why not try yoga or ayurveda as a last resort? I have nothing to lose." Many a times, yoga is the last resort after trying the conventional medical modality.

This was true of a lady that had severe sciatica nerve compression problem in her lower back. The musculoskeletal pain originated in her spine, plausibly from a herniated disc, and radiated down her leg. It hurt more when she walked. She had consulted an orthopedist and he had recommended vertebroplasty, a surgery for the herniated disc. This measure would cut out a bit of the lumbar disc above and/or below the nerve. Hopefully, it would take the pressure off the nerve.

A couple of days before her hip surgery she and her husband came into my yoga class and asked if I could help. (To qualify as yoga teacher from Kaivalydhama Yoga Institute, one has to be well-versed in human anatomy and physiology. This know-how is indeed valuable.) One common advice to all persons coming for Chikitsa is: please maintain a record of exercises, diets, and physical, mental and emotional changes that are clearly happening. I then advised her to consider all her options. She could try out some suggested physical exercises and mudras for a week or two. She should observe what is happening in her legs and hip joints, and see if there is any relief, meagre or meaningful, or if the pain is getting worse. Another suggestion made compulsively especially for overweight and obese persons is watch your weight, and cut out as much of fat, sugar and carbs as possible to bring down the weight to reasonable levels, viz., BMI (body mass index) lower than 25 or 24 if possible.

Even after days of simple and safe exercise, if there was no resolution of the sciatica problem, maybe she can see if medication and/or surgery could help. She tentatively accepted my yoga exercise regimen and some diet suggestions. Yoga persons don't make the call for surgery or otherwise. It is left to the intelligent patient to make the choice. Of her own volition she also postponed the vertebroplasty surgery after weighing the options. To learn from me the required yoga asanas (saral bhujangasana or sphinx, tadasana or palm tree pose, and a few other prone exercises without stressing the hip joints) she came to a modest one-hall Shiva temple in Global Mall, Norcross, GA which by the way did not have a special place for imparting and learning yoga. I took permission from the priest. Reluctantly he let me do the demo exercises for her in a corner of the hall. I also got her to repeat them in my presence so I could correct any mistakes. Her husband learnt them too so that he could help if need arose when she practiced the exercises at home. She home-practiced them morning and evening for a month. As expected, she got much relief from acute pain, and felt less pressure on the nerve. The pain persisted, but the nerve pinch was gone. The pain, she said, was mild enough to ignore. She was happy that she did not have the vertebroplasty surgery.

There is medical information to say that invasive interventions of that kind could be a) cumbersome b) painful c) unproductive, and d) the sciatica problem could revert as there is no guarantee it would go away for good and e) expensive like a big ticket item with a tab for at least $40,000 to $50,000 in America and about \$4000 to \$5000 in India. For the yoga training she received at HTA and the Global Mall Temple there was no cost to her, not a penny. A few months later, it was gratifying to see her come (actually burst) into my yoga class unexpected to pay her tributes to yoga training by bowing down.

The Case of Meniscus Tear

In another case, when an orthopedic surgeon suggested knee surgery to repair a professor's torn meniscus, the 70-year old, also a yoga teacher himself, exercised his options: He had heard and read that surgery for meniscus tear is often needless and wasteful especially if it is due to osteoarthritis. It would cost up to or more than \$10,000, not to speak of the potential harm it could wreck on the patient especially if the patient is a senior citizen. On account of arthritis, articular cartilage becomes less serviceable and surgery is virtually ineffective. In the teacher's case, it was not due to any arthritic snag, but due to a jerk caused by a pull when doing a rigorous dance at a religious celebration, *Radha Kalyanam*. And so there was some justification for surgery despite his age in the early Seventies. And yet, he did not opt for surgery and kept his own counsel. His yogic training told him to go gentle on heavy duty yogic exercises. He shed weight as part of the solution, though he was not overweight. He did simple non-rigorous yogic maneuvers, some in the form of mudras. Also gentle massages were resorted to.

He also sought chiropractic help. Critical to the healing process was also a vibrator table in the chiropractor clinic. He was asked to lie down on his back on a table in the clinic keeping the entire right leg and mainly the back of the knee on the vibrator table. The front knee was then covered with hot and cold towels, alternatively, for 30-35 minutes even as the back of the knee was getting a gentle quivering motion. After about 4 such sessions, and daily yoga exercises over a period of about 8 weeks, the tear in the meniscus healed up by itself. Full functionality of the knee returned and the professor was able to sit in vajrasana (sitting on folded knees, with upturned pointed toes at the back.) He could not tell any difference between before and after the meniscus tear. It was as if nothing had happened, except that some six months earlier when MRI was done, everyone could see the slit in the meniscus, and also see the ligaments somewhat threadbare or scruffy.

Today, even some seven years later, the the professor says that his knee works just fine letting him even jog or do the *utkatasana* or the chair posture without any fragility caused by the erstwhile torn meniscus. Of late there is increasing confirmation of the option available about knee surgery. There is a trend towards getting around knee surgery as the following excerpt from a TV show corroborates: The most common knee surgery is arthroscopic procedures for older patients. It is overprescribed because "….surgeons are treating patients in pain….Patients want options in treatment of their conditions, and fixes that might not always be realistic…..The data is conclusive, and surgery in this population is a cautionary tale."[25]

Lady with Breathing Issues

Once a lady oncologist brought her mother, perhaps around 76 to my yoga class, requesting me to teach deep abdominal breathing. To my surprise the mother had other health issues, not letting her sit in padmasana or lotus position on the floor on a mat. So I sat her on a chair, and sat myself in *vajrasana* on the floor doing the demo breathing. When I asked her to do simple breathing, I found she was fully into paradoxical breathing! In paradoxical breathing the abdomen looks like it is getting concave or sucked in while inhaling, and convex or inflating when exhaling. This is paradoxical because the stomach should be coming forward while inhaling and going in while exhaling. The lungs expand like a balloon with inhalation and contract with exhalation. Inhalation prods the diaphragm below the rib cage to move downward forward, convex to the spinal cord and later move in backward. She had problems unlearning that breathing. Under my guidance she kept practicing normal abdominal breathing for a while. Finally she learnt regular breathing. It was a pleasure to see the old woman normalize her breath, and even do deep abdominal breathing. The mother and daughter smiled happily as they left.

Cutting out Insulin Shots for Diabetes Type II

Then there is the case of an environmental engineer in his late forties. But for all practical purposes, he looked no more than in his early thirties and looked lean and skinny. His problem was diabetes Type II. He was administering himself insulin shots twice a day and taking medication. This was the reason he came to the HTA Yoga Class. His glycated hemoglobin A1C test gave out scores of 7 and anyone between 5.7 and 6.4 percent average blood sugar level is considered prediabetic. So he had passed that stage into diabetes. I prescribed several asanas that would massage his pancreatic cells and one of them was the *halasana* or the plough exercise. The engineer was advised to perform the asanas twice a day in the morning and in the evening. Some diet restrictions too were proposed such as consuming about two ounces of bitter gourd juice every morning, and cutting out sugar as much as possible. Also I told him not to smoke or drink alcohol if he did those.

It was not for another six months that I met him and by then I had forgotten all about him, except that he had consulted me. The moment he saw me he thanked me profusely but I did not connect with the circumstances that brought him to the yoga class. He recalled, for my benefit, what I had prescribed for his diabetes and how he vigorously followed the regimen. Week after week, he witnessed gradual improvements in his blood sugar levels. After a few months of this treatment, his A1C test gave him a score of 4.5 which is normal. He told me he had given up the insulin shots though he was still taking some Metformin medication in small doses.

At times the immune system gets to damage the beta cells in the pancreas and insulin output decreases. With this inadequate insulin production, diabetes sets in. Yoga appears to massage these cells and coax them to do their duty. In this case, YI seemed to be successful. Also see Chapter 13, Yoga and Diabetes.

Narrated above are just a few anecdotal cases that come to mind, but such cases are many, if not a legion including in mental health area. Getting yogic help for a health issue has been one of the minor reasons for learning yoga. Many that come to yoga, as we noted earlier, aspire to achieve the stamina, flexibility and robust health of athletes and sports professionals who apparently do what appear to be superhuman on the rugby, football or basketball courts like for example the incredible one-handed Emmanuel Hansel.

Temple Yoga

Yoga classes at the Hindu Temple of Atlanta got started early in 1992 when as a certified yoga instructor I found many devotees and visitors to the Temple with numerous ailments: arthritis, asthma, backache, cancer, diabetes, depression, heart diseases and hypertension, orthopedic ailments, obesity and others. Some came to learn just the breathing exercises because they were going to Badrinath, Kedarnath or Manasarovar and other high elevation places. The air density goes down, making oxygen scarcer, necessitating more breathing to get the same oxygen as at lower altitudes. Pranayama and other breathing exercises stand us in good stead at high elevations.

There were issueless couples seeking yogic remedies. Some young ladies had irregular monthly cycles and older ones had issues related to menopause. Pregnant ladies had learnt that yoga helps deliver babies without Caesarian sections, or an incision in the mother's abdomen. And their intention coming to yoga classes was to get that assurance of less arduous delivery of more healthy babies. Of course, a sizeable number just wanted to prevent future health problems and wanted to attain yogic fitness and wholesome health.

African-American Outreach

Much of this medical data about yoga students was received by way of volunteered information during casual post-yoga session conversations. About 15-20 percent of yoga learners have been medical professionals, including doctors and nurses. There were flight attendants from airlines (who have given me buddy passes!) and professors and dieticians from universities, as well as singers and dancers from the Temple's cultural activities besides university students. And over the last fifteen years, there has been large welcome increase in African-American persons, children in particular.

African-American men and women are part of the Temple outreach. They are a regular presence in yoga classes, with their children too coming to yoga class. The inner peace they attained doing yoga, they told me, was for them transcendental. At many classes, often they are the majority in the class. The Temple is delighted about helping out its outreach neighborhood. An African American enthusiast Chelsea Jackson who used to attend class at Temple Yoga appeared on the cover page of *Yoga Journal* a few years ago after attaining proficiency and starting her own classes and thus being one of the yoga pioneers in her community.

There are dozens of cases such as these without much documentation and case studies. African American progress in taking big strides in yoga learning has a salutary effect on societal health and wellness. Their performance of the asanas and exercises are often better than performance by some others.

Children have had separate classes. Initially they would monkey around laughing and giggling at the asanas and breathing exercises, but within a short time, got to be solemn and serious. Parents brought their children to make them focus better with yoga, and escape from attention deficit disorder (ADD) and attention deficit hyperactivity disorder (ADHD). They were looking for nonpharmacological solutions, without medications and their adverse side effects. There is amazing promise of rapid yoga education in children of all ethnicities, including Hispanic and A-A kids.

Many other yoga-related anecdotes outside of our yoga classes are in the public domain. Cancer victims, after trying out chemotherapy and radiation as well as surgery have come to ayurveda and yoga and have had miraculous results like becoming clinically clean after a bout of cancer. Amit Vaidya's case was mentioned earlier. The case of Dr. Timothy McCall MD and yoga expert, (acknowledged under Table 7 and again elsewhere) comes to mind and his narrative on how he handled his own lymph node cancer in his throat first with some ayurvedic relaxation and yoga is fascinating. Fuller description of this case is reported under Chapter 11 on Yoga and Cancer that follows.

Under the same Chapter there is also the case (study) of an oncologist at Sloan Kettering Memorial Cancer Institute, Dr. William Flowers who, as fate would have it, was diagnosed towards end of 1995 with colon cancer. He underwent conventional therapy of radiation and chemotherapy. There was a relapse two years later. Instead of going for any traditional cures he opted for yogic exercises which brought back the vital energy of his original life, galvanized him enough to see more cancer patients than before, contribute more research papers, spend more time with family and even go scuba-diving! The life extension due to yoga practice was perhaps about seven years for Dr. Flowers even in his terminal condition.

Alternative and Complementary Modalities

Regardless of what these positive and promising facts and statistics from clinical research and meta-analysis of clinical studies about YI may connote, the health care debate is presided over by professionals in the conventional modality. The conventional modality manages essentially all deliberations on health care. It has blazed new trails in human health and wellness. It has contributed to advance the scientific spirit in health care. There is little dispute about its enormous contribution to human welfare. However, what is being put forward is whether allopathy alone should do all the heavy-lifting and decision-making, and whether it can do it cost-effectively. Other health care modalities conceivably deserve a place at the health care table and decision-making. The other modalities have their areas of specialty. It may be a good idea to let them have the first shot at resolving a medical issues in their area of specialty.

This pattern of medical pecking order is perhaps as it should be in the West where there are no other worthwhile comprehensive medical modalities in health care. What could be a moot point is whether such an ecosystem is fully appropriate in India too, the home of ayurveda, yoga, siddha, unani and other indigenous systems, besides allopathy. Ayurveda and yoga are more than a couple of millennia old. Paradoxical as it may sound, they have older annals and chronicles than allopathy. The two main reasons for indifference towards alternate modalities could be a) Most of these modalities, till recently anyway, lacked a body of knowledge in the public domain about case studies, anecdotes, articles in peer reviewed journals, leave alone clinical trials to support claims. And b) At least in India colonial ways of decision-making in every domain of life persist especially given the ubiquitous western style of decision-making whether in administration, business, dress, education, entertainment, food, health care, medicine, transport or travel or any other.

Health care in India today is administrated, operated and worked by professionals belonging to the conventional medical profession. That ayurveda, siddha, unani and yoga manage to survive despite centuries of neglect speaks for itself about their value and infallible contributions to health and wellness. The practicing indigenous doctors are called Vaidya in ayurveda modality, Siddhar in siddha system, Hakim in unani medicine and Yogi or Vaidya in Medical Yoga. These doctors are simple and unassuming persons without any chip on their shoulders. Not all of them have documents of the medical profession. The physicians of other modalities did not have clinical trials at least till about five decades ago. They had no endorsements, no health insurance, and more often than not, no fees for their life-saving medications and treatments. There is the eminent case of the late oncologist Vaidya Sri Narayana Murthy, Shimoga, India achieving 70% success in curing cancer, offering consultation free with herbs and tree barks, a tradition in his family for 14 generations.[26] In 2016 the US National Cancer Institute tested thousands of plants and discovered Taxol, a potent anti-cancer drug in the bark of a tree. Taxol family of drugs is sold under the generic name Paclitaxel for up to $38 per dose.[27] Vaidya Narayana Murthy could have helped perhaps in all this endeavor.

Professional unassuming nature has cost indigenous doctors their seat at the health care discussion table, even in India. They are also often dismissed as quacks. It is a good augury that the AYUSH ministry in the Union government is trying to make good the neglect. But that seems is long way off despite respiratory (breathing) emergencies caused by COVID-19.

All modalities other than mainstream allopathy go by the name of alternative or complementary modalities. This sounds somewhat perplexing considering that yoga and ayurveda are several millennia older than allopathy and also more comprehensive and holistic. Allopathy, no doubt has the most modern and cutting edge instruments and protocols for diagnosing health problems. There are also random control trials (RCTs) for various medication and treatments under allopathy. What many in the health field are unaware is that the same scientific protocols and RCTs are becoming vogue in yoga, ayurveda, siddha and other complementary modalities, including homeopathy, which is the 'H' in the abbreviation AYUSH. More welcome is the fact that, of late, a new term is becoming commonplace: integrated medicine which is perhaps the beginnings of best practices in a true sense.

The ground realities are however, the same: all decision-making about all aspects of health care are by conventionally qualified physicians, many of whom may not have even known about alternative modalities and what they have in store to offer for health care. Thus it is not a surprise that yogic breathing mentioned above is rarely taught or prescribed in medical schools. Nor is it talked about even now at the height of the health crisis caused by Corona virus. There is a real need to foster integrated medicine through best practices selected on the basis of outcomes of clinical research. Western life styles too have contributed in no small measure to the eminence of allopathy with emphasis on treating symptoms and diseases with drugs, radiation, surgery and so forth rather than on preventing diseases in the first place, and of course bringing to bear a global view point, such as calling for lifestyle changes for lifestyle illness. Often there are alternative and complementary medicine or therapy including belly breathing, meditation, asanas, mudras and bandhas.

Major Causes of Death

In YVM it was originally intended to present the clinical evidence of outcomes of YI in the same order as the top ten causes of death. However, there are some departures from that order as detailed under 'Chapter Scheme'. The reason is there is urgency to present new evidence such as in the case of COVID-19 infections beleaguering mankind everywhere in the world. It was thus dealt with first. And so the order of presentation was broken. There is also some aptness in presenting the reader yoga-relevant facts that would provide the right contextual backdrop for presenting research facts about efficacy of YI. In the following pages diseases that are a major cause of death in the USA according to the Center for Disease Control and Prevention, and in India according to actuaries are listed together with the number of deaths or as percentage of total deaths so they can be ranked accordingly. Heart disease is absolutely at the top in both countries, followed by malignant neoplasms or cancer, accidents (mostly car-vehicle), respiratory diseases to which one could now add, COVID-19 deaths considering that the main medical issue with it is respiratory, shortness of breath, pleurisy and flue. This inference is easy to make despite the inconsistent information in the two tables below, the American data presented in actual numbers and Indian data in percentages.

Table 4: Top Ten Causes of death in 2017 in USA (COVID-19 not included)

Total Number of Deaths		
Rank	**All causes**	2,813,503
1	Diseases of heart	647,457
2	Malignant neoplasms or Cancerous tumors	599,108
3	Unintentional injuries	169,936
4	Chronic lower respiratory diseases	160,201
5	Cerebrovascular diseases	146,383
6	Alzheimer's disease	121,404
7	Diabetes mellitus	83,564
8	Influenza and pneumonia	55,672
9	Nephritis, nephrotic syndrome and nephrosis	50,633
10	Suicide	47,173

Source: Adapted from https://www.cdc.gov/nchs/data/hus/2018/006.pdf

Table 5: Top Ten Causes of Death in India (COVID-19 not included)

Rank	Cause of Death	% of Total Deaths (Ages 25-69)
1	Cardiovascular Diseases	24.8
2	Respiratory Diseases	10.2
3	Tuberculosis	10.1
4	Malignant and Other Tumors	9.4
5	Ill-Defined Conditions	5.3
6	Digestive Diseases	5.1
7	Diarrheal Diseases	5.0
8	Unintentional Injuries	4.6
9	Intentional Self-Harm	3.0
10	Malaria	2.8

Source: Adapted from https://life.futuregenerali.in/life-insurance-made-simple/cancer-heart-critical-illness-insurance/

What and how yoga can contribute to minimizing morbidities and mortalities described in the two tables above? The following chapters will address that question.

Chapter 2

Yoga and COVID-19

One of the most elemental mistakes committed by much of humanity is wrong breathing. Let us take this state of circumstances about SARS-COVID-19 which is *inter alia*, essentially a respiratory disease. There have been 117 million Corona virus cases in 219 countries and territories of the world and an alarming 2.6 million deaths as of March 07, This is 2.2 percent of COVID cases. Thanks to the new variants of the SARS-COV-2 virus, viz., B.1.1.7 (in UK), and B.1.351 (in South Africa), very soon there may be spikes in infections and mortality, the numbers going beyond 125 million infections and 3 million deaths, taking the casualty rate to 2.4 percent. New variant infections have been detected around the world.[28] There is fear of new waves in many parts of the world. There is an appalling and an avertable loss of human life. There is collateral loss in productivity, production, breakdowns in supply chains, extraordinary increases in unemployment, severe discontinuities in life, loss of business, government tax revenues, loss of wellness and unconceivable increases in health care costs, leave alone depression-like economic conditions. COVID-19 has also begotten much social, economic, educational, political as well as geopolitical strife, emergency, and dreadful conflict that is hastening the pace of history.

The symptoms of Corona Virus infection are: manifest shortness of breath and breathing problems, besides repeated chills, fever, sore throat, dry cough, dyspnea, diarrhea, headache, myalgia, body ache, loss of taste and smell, and so forth. There is acute respiratory agony. Here the classic breathing remedies of yoga could have a perceptible impact on COVID-19 patients. And what is regrettable is that much of this suffering could have been avoided by imparting speedily, basic yogic training especially in breathing, to as many willing people as possible anywhere in the world. Experts in medical yoga have also pleaded for the dissemination of yoga basics more widely to stem the Corona virus pandemic. Brief details are given below of this endeavor to press yoga into universal service to control as far as possible, the deleterious effect of COVID-19 to society which is making a mockery of health and well-being of even the high and mighty, prime ministers and presidents, leave alone the poor and the lay public.

Yoga and Corona Virus

Yoga offers classic breathing remedies that could have a perceptible impact on COVID-19 potential patients. More essentially, imparting training in yogic breathing practices will prevent the coronavirus disease in its severity. The modus flow chart of yoga influence on COVID is shown in the graphic below:

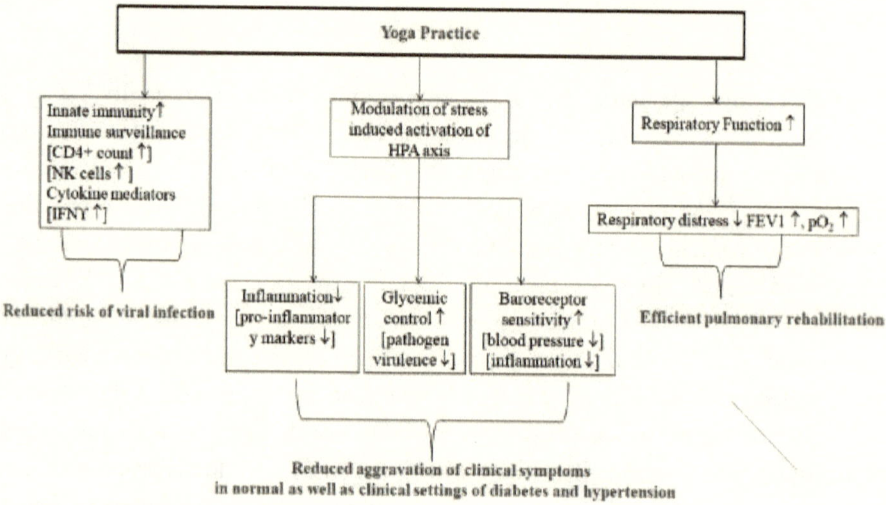

Fig.3: How Yoga Therapy Curbs COVID-19 Epidemic

Source: Nagarathna, R et al. "A Perspective on Yoga as a Preventive strategy for Coronavirus Disease 2019." International journal of yoga vol. 13, 2 (2020): 89-98. doi:10.4103/ijoy.IJOY_22_20 [29]

Nagarathna et al report of a significant improvement in PEFR (Peak Expiratory Flow Rate, measuring how fast a person can exhale) of over 20% within 30 minutes of breathing practice and with relief from acute airway obstruction. The sample size was 86 asthma patients who had breathing issues not dissimilar to those of Coronavirus. The intervention reduced panic and anxiety and helped participants in snapping out of the vicious cycle of aggravating bronchial obstruction. Similar results can be expected in cases of respiratory/pulmonary distress (shortness of breath) for Corona virus victims or those vulnerable to it. Also see Chapter 12 on Asthma and Yogic Breathing, p.125

The PEFR monitor is a hand-held instrument into which a person blows air as forcefully and as fully as possible. The PEFR scale is on the instrument itself and can be read off it. If the reading is between 80 – 100% of one's normal flow rate, it means that the person is normal and is in the green zone. If the reading is between 50 - 80%, it means that the breathing tubes are narrowing and some action may be needed to reverse the numbers. And if it goes down below 50 it means that the person is in the red zone and needs treatment. Age-specific yoga modules have been offered by Nagrathna et al..[30] A module of simple yoga exercises was suggested by VYASA's researchers and was used by hospitalized COVID-19 patients in Milano, Italy, where the health damage from COVID's first wave itself was frightening. One of the cardiac surgeons who was also a COVID-19 patient, reported to the authors: "We have reached scientific evidence that this simplified protocol sent by you is effective…."

COVID-19 Opinion Survey

In January 2021 this author conducted a quick opinion survey on WhatsApp of some sixty yoga students in Atlanta, GA who practice yoga regularly. The questions asked on WhatsApp were:

1. In this Coronavirus year 2020-21 how many of you practised yoga exercises regularly, that is about 4-5 days a week or more?
2. Did anyone of you experience Coronavirus symptoms or infection of COVID-19?
3. If so how many days did it take to get back to normal health?

The unanimous responses were:

1. All sixty students practiced yoga exercises including breathing exercises at least 4-5 days a week during 2020-21.
2. None of them got infected with the Coronavirus. One girl student, a beginner, had symptoms, but later came out Coronavirus negative. And she too later fell in line with the rest of the students.
3. There was no response to the third question for good reasons!

This is not a scientific sample survey, not random or cluster nor any other, but a convenient survey shedding light on what yoga could do, *ceteris paribus,* to the rest of America's or India's or world's population if only yoga was practised by them.

The convenient survey on WhatsApp above somewhat answered the question: Do practicing yogis fall sick with COVID 19 infection? Those that practice yoga regularly, almost daily, become less vulnerable to Coronavirus. The eventual complete answer would depend upon related factors: life styles, extent of exposure to stress factors, food consumption and diet, the degree of immune system compromise, standards of living, the yoga person's physical, economic, social, political, spiritual environment, mask-wearing behavior, social distancing, physical contact and interaction with members of family and of society, age, profession, workloads, and related factors. Despite these caveats, it is safe to take a broad view that the probability of a person practicing yoga regularly succumbing to Corona virus or similar infections, other things remaining the same, is much less than for a non-practicing lay man.

A large part of this exceptionalism of yoga can be attributable to its inward looking tendency. The yoga person activates his lymphatic nodes through exercises and thereby ensures that the immune system is geared to the serious job of instantly recognizing the intruding antigen riding on top of a pathogen of the virus. Cells specialize in producing antibodies and destroy the viral particles including the Coronavirus. It is as if she or he can see the virus mischief-maker trying to slip into the body, and being trounced by the cytokines released by the white blood cells.[31] Yoga perhaps helps in enabling the white blood cells not to overreact and let loose a cytokine storm which would complicate defense against the virus.

During the Coronavirus period it is possible that there is more pressure on some persons and expose them to more anxiety, fear and stress. The person not practicing yoga would by default invoke the sympathetic nervous system and expose such nervous system to daily hammerings by stress events including fears about the virus. This would exacerbate wear and tear of body and mind, and of the cohesive human. The yoga person on the other hand would invoke the parasympathetic nervous system to respond to familiar 'fight or flight' anxiety and stress settings, and situations in daily life. The yogi would resort to invoking the PNS, and the non-activation of H-P-A axis. This would keep the Corona virus under control and help the immune cells to expedite their elimination. Breathing practices under yoga alone would almost completely eliminate the need for ventilators to pump air into lungs.

Yoga's Potential to Save Trillions

It can be speculated, if not postulated that if only a quarter of the Corona virus infected persons knew the basics of yogic deep abdominal breathing called pranayama, and bellows or bhastrika (forced and quick exhalations), a) those infected would have had a much higher probability of recovering faster, b) the resort to ventilators would have been much less, c) mortality rates would have been substantially less than what they have been. And d) the loss of resources would have been much less than what was expended. The economies would have chugged along faster, with much less loss of productivity and production. World over, overall losses could have been trimmed down by trillions of dollars. In contrast, the cost of imparting this basic training in breathing and related exercises would not have been more than a fraction of a fraction of all this spanking loss. And yet, public health messages are not there, not even in India, urging all people to learn to take to deep abdominal breathing like in pranayama, and make it their default breathing. It is to be expected that such messages often fall on deaf ears, especially of those with rugged individualism that gets better of their commonsense. And also yoga is still not yet prevalent enough as a champion curer of respiratory diseases. The same could be true of a small minority in the medical field with some aversion towards yoga and alternative modalities, and also wanting to protect their turfs.

AYUSH Protocol for Treatment of Corona Virus

In the background of the Corona pandemic, the AYUSH Ministry, Government of India has come up with a yoga-ayurveda based National Clinical Management Protocol giving clear guidelines to professionals in yoga and ayurveda on the treatment of the infection in different stages of the disease. Such guidelines would provide uniformity and consistency in the treatment. The Government believes that the protocol would end ambiguity about Ayurveda and Yoga-based solutions for the clinical management of Covid- 19. The subsequent versions of the Protocol will cover other disciplines of Ayush. What is heartening, the public will have access to these solutions and reduce the hardships brought in by the pandemic. In the formulation of the common solutions protocol, expert committees from national institutes and Central Council for Research Centers have collaborated to craft the protocol for the management of Covid-19.[32] It is already April 2021 and one does not still see the alternative modalities in play anywhere. The rage is all about the vaccination to put a stop to Coronavirus or at least stymie it.

Chapter 3

Yoga and Health Care Costs

A health care modality's efficacy in curing a health condition or in preventing it is a significant factor for its wider practice. Along with that, the cost-effectiveness is also a consideration. America is known to have the most expensive health care system in the world, and yet, it is a moot point if it is the most efficient or the most cost-effective one. The data on which the graph in Fig. 4 on Yoga Impact on American Health Care Costs, is created, is itself based on the fact that the per capita health care spending in the US was almost $10,739 or a total of $3.7 trillion in 2017. From these statistics we estimated that the US population was put at 326 million in 2017.

Assuming the trend line trajectory continues, savings in health care costs due to increased number of Americans taking to yoga would exceed $1 trillion by 2025. Both physical and mental health issues are being tackled successfully by yoga modality, and if decision-makers give it a larger mandate than at present, with just minimal increases in facilities for imparting yoga instruction to millions more, the wellness scenario in America can be transformed into a more rational stratagem with much less of Alzheimer's, asthma, backaches, cardiac illness, cancer, dementia, diabetes, pneumonia, anxiety and stress-caused mental illness, attention deficit disorder, drug addiction, and many others. If there is more prevalence of rational decision-making, with increased resort to yogic solutions, if not yogic way of life, especially in mental health care, it would be possible to get ambitious about reducing health care costs more drastically and bring them on par with those of other advanced countries like Canada, UK, France, Germany and their like. And may be do even better.

In India, there is much more awareness of what yoga is and what it promises, but there is a wide gap between awareness and practice. Thus, for example, out of 101,643 persons in rural areas all over India who participated in a yoga awareness poll, 94,135 or 92.6% believed that yoga helped improved life style. Similarly out of 98,518 who responded to a question about yoga and diabetes, 90102 or 91.5% believed that yoga could help with diabetes. But the actual number of persons who took to yoga practice was a despicable 12%, far disproportionate to the number believing in yoga.[33] In America one could guess that the gap between those that are aware of yoga benefits and those that actually practice it, is narrower, considering the smaller size of the population as well as the larger number of well-informed persons compared to India.

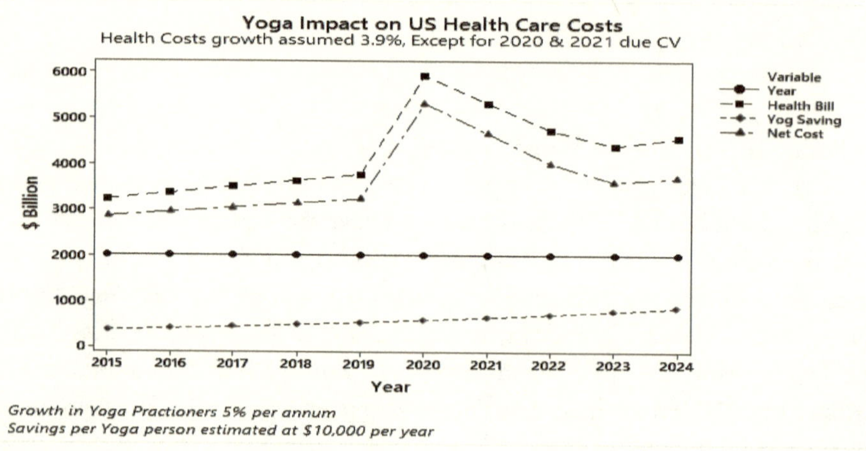

Fig 4: Yoga Impact on US Health Care Cost

Source: S. Char 2020

Fig. 5 presents per capita health care cost data age-wise for different advanced countries. The US curve is way above those of other countries for all ages, in particular those in the age groups 35 and above.

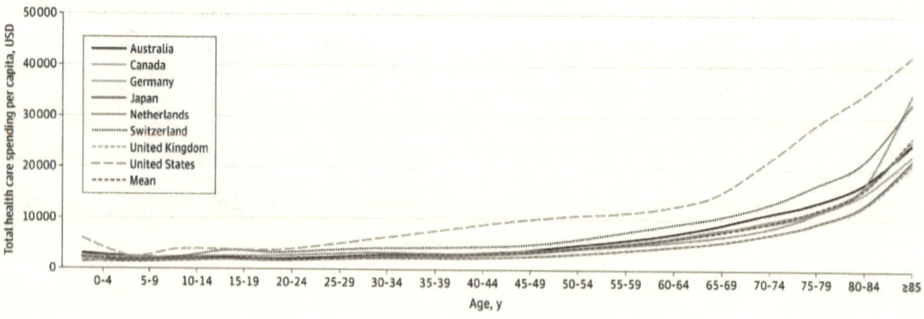

Fig.5: Per Capita Health Care Costs in 8 Advanced Countries

Source: JAMA Netw Open. 2020; 3(8):e2014688. doi:10.1001/jamanetworkopen.2020.14688
Spending is purchasing power parity–adjusted. The mean includes all countries except the US.

Yoga Practice and Healthcare Costs

It is common knowledge that while much is being done to ameliorate sickness and improve health standards of the living, there is sizeable waste in health care everywhere. One reason is not taking account of what results of clinical tests prove about yoga capabilities. Evidence-based deployment of yoga techniques for illness, particularly those in the area of mental health cannot wait further. This suggestion is made to improve the health outcomes as well as to make health care more cost-effective. Second, the prices of pharmaceuticals and of treatment are much higher than anywhere, including across the border in Canada or Mexico. The cost of medical services are about 5 to 10 times more expensive than elsewhere. There is much evidence of inflated charges for treatment of most diseases. What cannot be denied is that taxes paid in Europe in countries like Britain, France, and others are higher than in the USA. However, it is a moot point if universal health coverage would cause taxes paid in USA to go up except marginally. In America one has to buy medical insurance from the health insurance companies or the government at a relatively high premium. People also have to pay compulsory Medicare insurance tax, deducted from one's payroll, while in service or working, to fund the somewhat free health care coverage after retirement at age 65. There is Medicare A, B, C, D and even all the way till G. This array of multiple coverage caters to the fears of millions of Americans that are scared stiff of a) inevitably falling sick with one or the other sickness and b) with insurance premium payments suddenly becoming inadequate to cover a new little twist to a sickness like arthrtis, backache, cancer, diabetes, or hypertension.

There is broad agreement that health care waste could account for about 30 to 35% of health care expenditures. These are conservative estimates. And yet there is something like the Fermi Paradox about such savings in expenditures not materializing. There is ample evidence of extraterrestrial or ET intelligence in the universe, but no one has encountered or seen such ETs! [34,35] This is the Fermi paradox! Despite numerous efforts made, including the passing of the Affordable Care Act (Obamacare) 2010, there is little flattening of the uptrend in the trend line portraying Health Care expenditure. Even as the GDP is going up, so is the Health Care cost as a percentage of GDP.

Peer-reviewed gray literature giving evidence for the 2012-19 period came up with the following causes and estimates of the ranges of wastes. The dollar figures given next to such range of wastes is the savings from measures to eliminate or address such excess. The range of waste and excesses is estimated at $760 billion to $935 billion. Savings from interventions, excluding savings from administrative complexity, was put at \$191 billion to \$286 billion, representing a potential 25% reduction in the total cost of waste. A more thorough estimation of waste including in Medicare would easily pierce the trillion dollar mark.

Table 6: Waste in US Health Care Expenditure

SIX DOMAINS OF WASTE IN HEALTH CARE EXPENDITURE	
Failure of care delivery, \$102.4 B to \$165.7 B;	Possible Savings: \$44.4 B to \$97.3 B
Failure of care coordination, \$27.2 B to \$78.2 B;	Possible Savings: \$29.6 B to \$38.2 B;
Overtreatment \$75.7 B to \$101.2 B;	Possible Savings: \$12.8 B to \$28.6 B;
Pricing failure, \$230.7 B to \$240.5 B;	Possible Savings: \$81.4 B to \$91.2 B;
Fraud and abuse, \$58.5 B to \$83.9 B;	Possible Savings: \$22.8 B to 30.8B.
Administrative complexity, \$265.6 Billion.	Possible Savings: Nothing mentioned

Source: Compiled by author from Institute of Medicine, Berwick MB and Hackbarth (JAMA editorial)

These costs are exclusive of Administrative costs. Administrative costs per capita are far in excess of similar costs in other advanced countries. This is shown in Fig.6.

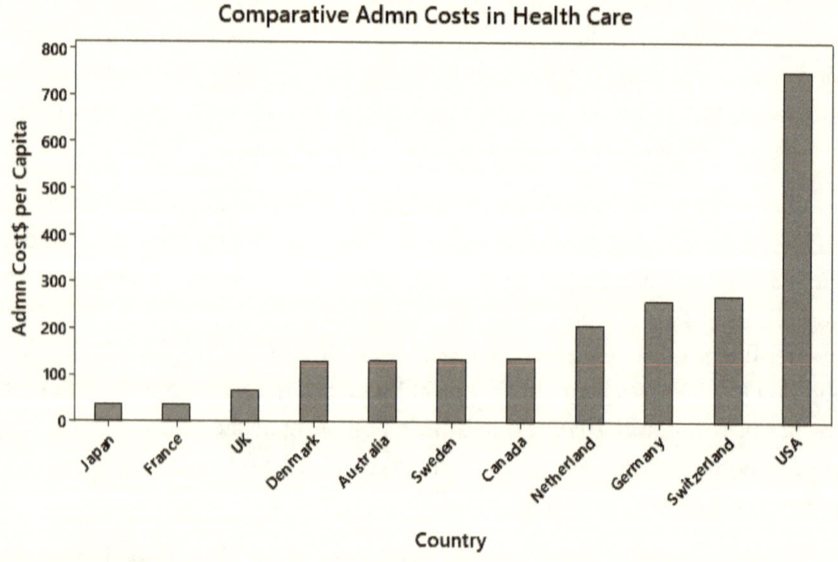

Source: Data from JAMA

Fig 6: Comparative Administrative Costs in Advanced Countries. For details see: Bauchner H, Fontanarosa PB. Health Care Spending in the United States Compared With 10 Other High-Income Countries: What Uwe Reinhardt Might Have Said. JAMA. 2018;319(10):990–992. doi:10.1001/jama.2018.1879

Chapter 4

Yoga and Health Care Discussion

In today's national health care discussions there is such an exhaustive coverage of health related issues that it would be logical to conclude that all issues relevant to healthcare are being discussed and all stakeholders in health care and wellness are represented. This is not true. Not all modalities are represented nor are all stakeholders have a say even edgeways! Yoga practioners are virtually disenfranchised although there is ample evidence of the efficacy of yoga modality, not just as a preventive or prophylactic, but even as therapeutic medicine. If there is more awareness of the capabilities of yoga as a remedial modality in its own right, it does not show up in practical terms as prescribed exercises for patients. Instead of just 14 million prescriptions in 2014 as noted earlier, there should have been at least several times that many.

There is increasing talk of outcomes of yoga interventions at various meetings of top American medical schools.[36] However, when push comes to shove, like in the present juncture of COVID 19 infections, when there is desperate search for new medicines and vaccines for it, there is hardly any mention, leave alone candid discussion about the need to boost nonpharmacological modalities, to boost the immune system or the lymph nodes, to calm the mind of panicking public, employing proven yogic methods. This is the backdrop for coming up with the following five ignored aspects of health care in America and more so in India, the very home of yoga.

Five Key Yoga Points and Public Health

There are five reasons for yoga remaining in the backwash of health care and not in the mainstream.

First, people that believe in self-care and think that individuals themselves are responsible to a large extent for their own well-being, for their wellness and health, and not the Government, not legislators/congressmen, the bureaucrats, the insurers, not even the physicians, have little representation in this crucial discussion of healthcare. It's time yoga practioners are heard! That would also help yoga play a more useful role in health care deliberations whether in India or America, or anywhere else.

Simple but regular work-outs prevent yoga persons from falling sick. Beyond standard wellness, these routines help us enjoy vigorous health; meaning not just lack of sickness but an ability to cope with stress, stay energetic, radiate health and spread good cheer around. Some yoga persons maintain enviable health without taking medications, perhaps not even aspirin. Such persons in the health insurance pool are the hedge against the outsized dollar drains caused by patients with serious cardiac problems, cancer, dialysis users, ER users, and others that often need to resort to both routine and upscale treatments.

Health Insurers, including Medicare, should be beseeching people who are yoga-knowledgeable expert health promoters to join the discussion of how to make the health care system more effective and also reduce these ongoing, expensive claims. They should be interviewing persons from other modalities on the evening TV news about how yoga practioners hardly spend the nation's health insurance money, and how more people can be trained to become responsible for promoting their own health. Health care policy makers need to hear how all can benefit from yoga practioners who do exercises regularly, do not fall sick and therefore do not make too many outsize insurance claims. If health care policy makers learn more about these real possibilities, they would take steps to increase the number of yoga coaches and mentors and also yoga practioners.

However just the opposite is happening. Unfortunately, wholesome health gained from yoga has made yoga persons actually outliers to the health discussions, and their views are deemed irrelevant to the health care deliberations. They are beyond practical. The people who do figure prominently in decision making on health matters, are the ones driving up healthcare costs. These discussions are targeted at the "typical" 50 and over, who take some medication or the other, pop some capsule, pill, or tablet, inject insulin, or indulge in combinations thereof; and likely they would have had some heart, kidney, or cancer surgery or some other frailty or invasive procedure. Views of people who consistently exercise, who take responsibility for prophylactic measures and protocols, are not present in these deliberations. They have been graduated and measured off.

Second, there is no natural law all people fall sick the same time. There is no deterministic certainty of a majority of persons falling sick in any one time dimension. This is the assumption underlying universal health care (UHC) coverage for uninsured persons under the Affordable Care Act. UHC or Medicaid for all is considered impractical because it implies that every one of the 340 million Americans, or a good majority of them, is unavoidably going to be sick at the same time; and the system will become despicably overloaded, and will crash, like at the peak of the COVID-19 emergency when there were no adequate beds or ventilators in New York hospitals for infected persons. On the other hand it is equally possible for the health conscious to be deterministic in a positive way.

Yoga practioners have alliances like the Yoga Alliance and the International Association of Yoga Therapists. These groups have a demonstration effect on a sizable, well-informed population. Groups could show what a purposeful life is, how life style and diet modifications can be practically done, like eschewing smoking, alcoholic beverages, drugs, and avoiding unhygienic practices including animal-based food besides minimizing fat, sugar and carbs. Yoga groups of this kind could have considerable weight as a force for effective therapy and cost-effectiveness. And yet there are entrenched positions taken by conventional medical systems making it hard for yoga to contribute its humble two bits to health care.

Standing on one's own feet, is, fair and square in accordance with the belief of two radically different leaders: the objectivist that did not want to live for others, Ayn Rand and champion of black rights and autonomy, Malcolm X. They both wanted people to be fiercely independent of governments in matters like health and nothing else than yoga can help achieve their objective of self-dependence in health care.

In India, for the indigent the Government has brought out the Ayushman Bharat Pradhan Mantri Jan Yojana AP-PMJAY mentioned on page 2-3. Under this scheme, the Government offers financial help of up to Rs. 5 lakhs per family per year for secondary and tertiary care hospitalization to over 107.4 million poor and vulnerable families which is about 530 million beneficiaries. While this could be the right thing to do, a yoga or a ayurveda person would be curious to learn what part of the Government health budget is being spent on educating the public about ayurveda or yoga's effective prophylactics and cures in the form of simple breathing and physical exercises? Will not the offer of Rs. 5 lakhs, by itself, induce the indigent to make impulsive choices and discourage them from discovering the goodness of yoga cures? Is this not like the same complacency or the Peltzman effect generated by a seat-belt to a rash car driver? This is very likely to occur in the absence of a vigorous health education campaign, in the absence of which there will be very few takers for ayurveda or yoga. Laidback health insurance with no push for indigenous modalities will marginalize them.

Third, the effectiveness of yoga intervention has been known for some time and a large body of research data has been compiled. However, all that useful data is not effortlessly available. Much of the research, for example at Indian research institutions like Kaivalyadhama, VYASA, Krishnamacharya Yoga Mandiram, Morarji Desai National Institute of Yoga (MDNIY), All India Institute of Medical Sciences, and many others are virtually not accessible in India or abroad. These yoga research organizations are like separate islands of research and not very well-known in America, Europe and non-English speaking world. They may have institutional research journals, but they are not known to the lay public. They are not mentioned in peer-reviewed journals and this could be on account of the somewhat laborious protocols the journals follow, to comply with which the research institutions may not have all the wherewithal. One of the rationale for YVM is to make good this gap. However, that is just a miniscule effort in English language, when there is urgent need for Hindi and vernacular YVM, not to speak of Spanish, French and other YVM for the world.

Like the details in Table 1 about conditions that were helped by yoga in Britain, given below are results of an earlier British survey showing medical conditions helped by yoga. There is critical need for similar surveys in India and other countries. A survey of 2,700 persons conducted by the Yoga Biomedical Trust, London, came up with data below:

Table 7: Medical Conditions Helped by Yoga

Medical Condition	Number of people Reporting	Percentage Helped by Yoga
Alcoholism	26	100
Anxiety	838	94
Arthritis and Rheumatism	589	90
Asthma or Bronchitis	226	88
Back Disorders	1142	98
Cancer	29	90
Diabetes	10	80
Duodenal Ulcers	40	90
Heart Disease	50	94
Hemorrhoids	391	88
High Blood Pressure	150	84
Insomnia	542	82
Menopausal disorders	247	83

Medical Condition	Number of people Reporting	Percentage Helped by Yoga
Menstrual Problems	317	68
Migraine	464	80
Neurological and Neuromuscular Diseases	112	96
Obesity	240	74
Premenstrual Syndrome	848	77
Smoking	219	74

Source: The Yoga Biomedical Trust, London, reproduced from "Yoga as Medicine", by Timothy McCall, M.D. (2007), p.5.

The ironic fact is that yoga has been helping human beings to enjoy complete holistic fitness and also cure numerous physiological and mental health issues for a few thousand years. However they are not documented as per the protocols and procedures of the current system of clinical research with experimental and control groups, random clinical trials (RCTs), meta-analysis, Cochrane Review Assessment of previous trials under a meta-analysis, and sophisticated statistical assessments. They may be just Simple Simon pre and post analysis, with student t test results, Chi-Square tests, ANOVA, Independent Sample Tests like Levene tests and so forth. Where the data distributions are not bell-shaped there may be use of nonparametric tests like Wilcoxon, or Mann-Whitney. All this is followed by discussion and other health care modalities need to follow the methods of the dominant modality in order to establish their credentials and make progress. It is a good omen that research developments in this direction have been already afoot and in the works for a few decades.

There are sea changes in current research in alternative and complementary modalities. Some of the recent data and statistical analyses in India are one up on research elsewhere. Included in the references for this publication are a few of these. Hopefully the recent research works may have a different reception. They are already part of the eminent databases such as Cochrane Library, Medline, Embase, Access Medicine, PubMed, Clinical Key and several others. They are also in the limelight of bibliographic citations of National Institute of Health (NIH), National Center for Complementary and Integral Health (NCCIH), and similar research institutions. British journals such as Lancet, British Medical Journal and many others are recognizing yoga research in India and elsewhere.

Fourth, last mile delivery of important public health messages such as smoking is hazardous to health has reached the designated audiences and also having sound health effects except among persons that are deniers and/or defiant. However, many other educational messages don't seem to be reaching the target audiences such as better use of complementary or alternative modalities for health care. NIH website: 'Yoga, What You Need to Know, What is Yoga and How Does it Work' accessible at *https://www.nccih.nih.gov/health/yoga-what-you-need-to-know* is a good beginning. Public health messages about the vital need to hand wash, wear masks and social distance from one another during COVID-19 have reached home. There are however highly libertarian individualistic groups that believe in defying them. Hopefully this messaging would continue. They are particularly needed in communities where there is social and economic decline, Skid-Row mindsets, unhealthy work places, and where there is customary resort to perilous addictive drugs and drinks.

Campaigns are also needed to make good the lack of awareness of the fact that the human body is an extraordinary bio-chemical factory that has a physiological process called homeostasis that self corrects often without (excess) medications. Case studies could show how homeostasis can be aided and furthered by yoga, how meditation and deep abdominal breathing can help with asthma, apnea and other breathing problems, over-weight, obesity and many others.

Fifth, people make life style changes when there is a tangible incentive. It should be irresistible for choosing healthy habits, such as lower premiums for event-free wellness periods. This kind of incentive is used for other forms of insurance, such as vehicle insurance. Publicizing positive news induces other languid persons also to comply. This has worked in taxation. When Britain recently announced how the annual tax returns have been filed on or before time by a majority of tax payers, other laidback tax payers dragging feet got alerted and started falling in line. Many European countries are motivating change in healthcare this way as well. What is sauce for the goose is sauce for the gander. Let Indians, Americans and all else too have those incentives for self-promotion of robust health and wellness.

Chapter 5

Yoga and the Mind

One of the main contributions of yoga and ayurveda to the fundamentals of diagnostics is their age old breakthrough discovery that agitated and troubled minds are the generic triggers for numerous illnesses of the mind, the heart, the respiratory system, the digestive system, the central nervous system and of other parts of the human body. Exceptions are infectious diseases like fevers, the corona virus and their like, and congenital diseases. Even in such cases, enough evidence has been adduced to reveal the contribution of yogic practices to bring down the probability of getting sick by boosting the immune system and otherwise down- or upregulating phenotype or the gene expression, minimizing gene-related hassle.

In *Yoga Vasishtha,* Rama, the hero of the ancient epic Ramayana asks his Guru and Sage, Vasishtha: what is the origin of mental and bodily diseases? Vasishtha responds that the illnesses of the body are secondary, and the afflictions of the mind are primary. Many an illness has its origin in the mind. This ranking of mental illness over that of the body is based on the scientific understanding that in the matter of disease-causation, the mind looms over the body. Often instincts like desire and egotism look up to the mind as their home, and prompt the body to perform karmas or acts not congenial for the wellness of the mind or the body.

Guru Vasishtha continues that when a person's mind is agitated, the Prana vaayu (the normal abdominal breath, the life energy force) of the person decays into an irregular pattern. The distressed person is a like an animal hit by an arrow, staggering on its walk with little self-control.[37] Such a person would be vulnerable to any illness, and with a weakened immune system would be at risk for any infection.

This is remarkable insight in modern medicine: the brain's transactions and reactions to events and one's own ideas, propel a person's self or Aham (the I in terms of personality) as an entity. Any disapproval of one's ideas stokes tension and triggers numerous reactions which could lead to chronic anxieties and stress which are predatory, even if in an overstated, but otherwise true sense. Yoga's specialty is one of channeling tension to the parasympathetic nervous system instead of making the sympathetic nervous system bear the brunt of all tension. In other words nervousness is handled biomechanically, like second nature, sparing the latter of much of the bulldozing pressure of tension. The wear and tear on the system is thus minimized. Enter GABA, the gamma aminobutyric acid.

The Amazing Human Brain

Sage Vasishtha taught Rama, his most eminent pupil, as earlier observed, that most of the health and wellness problems have our mind as their source. The mind's output of electrical impulses, ideas or brainwaves are not always in harmony with the guidelines or parameters of health and wellness. In the pursuit of instantaneous gratification and happiness, there is always a tendency to go for an excess of good things of life, examples: food and leisure, and avoid even a bare minimum of hard choices of life, like being self-controlled, well-organized and choosing wholesome living, examples: self-reflection to improve oneself constantly or practicing objectivity.

Contrary to the deep-rooted belief that the heart is the seat of emotions, it is certain parts of the brain such as the thalamus and hypothalamus that are linked to emotions and the reactions to events and happenings. The amygdala, almond-shaped organs on either side of the brain, are regarded as fear processing and emotional center of the brain. The amygdala twins, one on each side of the brain, are the epicenter of feelings and sentiments as well as the organs that literally and figuratively make up our mind about 'fight or fight' options when potential threats loom large on the horizon. Orders go forth from them to increase the breath and heart rates to prepare the entire human being to handle the impending peril.

The brain weighs just about three pounds or about 2% of human body weight, but consumes disproportionately more oxygen and calories such as 20% of the total. 73% of the brain is all water. It is home to some 100 billion neurons. Neurotransmission is the interaction and communications of the neurons that results in the generation of thoughts. The gap between two neurons is called a synapse. When communications between two neurons over the synaptic cleft occur it is called a neurotransmission. Such transmission takes place through a process of exocytosis or the release of communicative biomaterial and its capture by another neuron through a process of endocytosis. The smallest unit of a thought is a bioelectrical impulse. When millions of such impulses get melded, they may become thoughts.

It is not yet scientifically proven that something like lateralization of brain functions occur in the left and the right hemispheres of the brain. There is the left-brain or right-brain dominance. It is believed that the left brain hemisphere is the center for logical functions, intelligence, mathematical critical thinking and allied analyses whereas the right brain is more a seat of emotions, judgement, and so forth. The two hemispheres are linked by the corpus callosum, a C-shaped bundle of nerve fibers under the cerebral cortex. There is agreement that while these could be broadly true, there is no specialization and both hemispheres collaborate and work out together. It is correct to say that the jury is still out on this.

Brain Functions Improved by Yoga Practice

Yoga is known to stimulate brain activity. Supporting this conclusion is the 2015 study[38] that proficiently examined the impact of yoga practice on cognitive capability on 30 normal engineering students. The students were randomly selected into yoga group and a control group. The yoga group performed yoga for 90 minutes, six days a week for a duration of five months. The impact was to be assessed using electroencephalograph (EEG) band powers. The yoga practising group recorded increased α, β, and δ EEG band powers and significant reduction in θ and γ band powers. Increased α and β power are indicative of enhanced cognitive functions such as for example memory and concentration whereas δ represents higher degree of synchronization of brain activity. There was a decrease in the heart rate index meaning a more efficient heart function and better cardiovascular fitness like in the case of an athlete. Comprehension and perception increased, as measured by the neural activity index β/θ.

Other gains from yoga practice included increase in attention resource index, a decrease in executive load index and a decrease in the ratio. Physiologically, there was an increase in heart rate variability, increased SDNN/RMSSD and a reduction in LF/HF ratio. The overall conclusion of the study was that there were significant improvements in various cognitive functions. These functions include performance enhancement, neural activity, attention, and executive function. Stress management improved with more resort to parasympathetic nervous system activity, and balanced autonomic nervous system reactivity.

The four brain chemicals that make one happy are mentioned below: **DOSE: dopamine** that just helps anticipate a happy event and makes us happy, **oxytocin** considered the love hormone that make us feel like friends, **serotonin** in our guts that signals hunger and **endorphins** that boost energy when needed as during a 'fight or flight' situation. It is this biochemical that prods and empowers the marathon runner in a competitive race instead of entertaining ideas to drop out due to fatigue or ennui. Some emotions like love can affect our health and wellbeing considerably, whereas rage and fury could impact us in the opposite way. Yoga's specialty is restoration of equanimity of the mind which by itself does not leave much latitude or room for agitations and anxieties. With such solid stability and resilience, the mind and body are able to successfully take on any major, leave alone minor, health challenge. For this success to come to pass, the human, the owner of the mind-body, needs to be an enabler, letting the faculties of the body and mind function to their full proficiency and investing much trust in them. He or she needs this resolve, grit, strength of character, or all three rolled into one: *sankalpa* to make progress along rock-hard wellness.

There is no dearth of clinical studies about yoga treatment for mental health issues such as anxiety, depression, panic, stress and trauma. A 2020 review of 27 studies relating to anxiety and stress among youth (age below 18 years) was carried out to evaluate the implementation and effectiveness of yoga postures for reduction of symptoms relating to these two mental health concerns. Thorough search was done to put together all studies up to November 2018 relating to yoga intervention in experimental studies of youth having symptoms of anxiety and depression. Heterogeneity in the types of exercises from the yoga package such as asanas (which ones?), mudras (which ones?), breathing exercises, bandhas and so forth) was common impacting the efficacy of the interventions. This situation arises because many a time the kind of YI used is not clarified or mentioned in sufficient detail. Let us say mudras and breathing were used in a particular YI. The researcher cannot tell from this data whether Bhastrika or Kapalabhati was used in breathing, or it was nadishodana pranayama or *viloma/pratiloma* and so forth. The same applies for mudras: what mudra was used – *bhoochari, bhujangini, kaki, shanmukhi* or any other. Some are simple or others more complicated. Heterogeneity also happens due to inexactness about doses (how many times a day or week the exercises were done?), comorbidities of patients, ethnic diversity, cultural differences impacting life styles, and so forth. High values for heterogeneity such as 75 to 90%, or even lower, make it difficult to generalize results or apply for specific situations.

The reviewers synthesized the required information extracted from the studies. Overall 70% of the studies showed improvements. 58% of the studies showed reduction in symptoms of both anxiety and depression. Anxiety symptoms alone came down in 25% of studies. 70% of the studies dealing only with anxiety showed improvements and in the case of studies that dealt with depression alone, 40% showed changes for the better.[39]

The overall effect of much of this yoga package is the generation of gamma aminobutyric acid (GABA) with a molecular chemical formula of $C_4H_9NO_2$.

(Fuller account of GABA on page 64). This is a neuro-inhibitor spreading GABA on neurons and holding back or slowing down inter-neuron communications. Thus it serves as a pacifier and ends neuro-chatter. The vagal tone is improved. The autonomic parasympathetic nervous system (PNS) kicks in. The PNS manages body physiology when the conscious mind is at rest. The explanation about GABA makes it easier to follow yoga's physiological and neurological mechanism for remedying problems.

Yoga and Migraine Headaches

For a granular description of the ordeal that migraine victims go through read Lauren Collins' narration of Cindy McCain's headache misery. It unerringly informs how this "disability" badgers its prey. Cindy did not have much success with any treatment including Botox. As a result, in her address to the American Headache Society (AHS) the much exasperated Cindy says "I will do anything including chewing broken glass if it would help me get rid of this."[40] Stress and migraines feed on each other in a vicious cycle: more stress causes more migraines which in turn cause more stress, and thus they try to propagate themselves. Even reduction in stress, paradoxically, causes migraines! Each person's stressor trigger for migraines could be different. There is a characteristic feeling or sensation before the onset of migraines.

There are differences between plain headaches and migraines, though both have their origin in stressful situations. Headaches are mild and can hurt on both sides of the forehead, and migraines are usually throbbing intense pains on one side of the forehead. They are episodic. Other symptoms of migraines are dizziness, nausea, blind spots or flashing lights.[41] Allergic sinusitis with a runny nose could cause a headache, but it may not be migraine. But you cannot vouch for it, and sinusitis could be common to both headaches.[42] AHS states some two thirds of chronic migraine sufferers have insomnia issues and do not get to have their full quota of sleep and rest.

AHA offers behavioral therapy for this condition so patients may sleep better.[43] This includes relaxation training, yoga's formidable strong suit. Plain headaches are not debilitating like migraines. But both are unwelcome aches that can impede productivity and initiatives. 85% of chronic migraine sufferers are women in the age group of 25-55 years. Migraines are episodic neurological disorders often triggered absurdly enough by mild phenomena like sudden drop in barometric pressure, changes in intensity of light and sound, some foods including excess caffeine, perfumes, stress and tension, inadequate sleep, smells, and even inherited genes. It could also occur because of overconsuming prescribed medication for such headaches, believing more is better. New evidence shows that 80 percent of migraine cases are due to stress.[44] Chronic stage of migraine is when a person suffers it 15 days or more in a month.

To come to think of stress, this beast, also incarnating itself as anxiety and tension, is culpable for 70 to 80 percent of human health afflictions including the main causes of death, viz., heart illnesses, cancer, unintentional injuries and accidents, diabetes, respiratory diseases (under which you can now bring in COVID-19) and numerous others. To be effective, therapy for migraines must match the beast's overpowering muscle. The treatment should include prophylactic life style changes, which alas, are the most difficult to modify for many people. For migraines specifically, Yoga guru, BKS Iyengar has prescribed 18 yogic exercises including breathing exercises. About half of them involve forward bending like in Veerasana with a crepe bandage around the eyes.[45]

Clinical studies of Yoga therapy for migraine headache has yielded encouraging results as shown. A 2007 clinical study of Yoga Intervention (YI) with a randomized control trial design for migraine management at University of Rajasthan (UofR) reported that YI brought about significant reduction in frequency of migraine headaches in patients.[46] The study had a sample of 72 patients with migraine without aura and they were randomly assigned to yoga therapy group or self-care group for a 3-month period. The patients maintained a headache diary in which they recorded the severity of headache (on a 0-10 scale) and the nature of the pain component as per McGill pain questionnaire. There were recordings of anxiety as per the Hospital anxiety depression scale as well as a recording of the medication.

The results of the UofR study brought out the efficacy of YI: After adjustment for baseline values, the migraine complaints relating to a) headache intensity ($P < .001$), b) frequency ($P < .001$), c) pain rating index ($P < .001$), d) affective pain rating index ($P < .001$), e) total pain rating index ($P < .001$), f) anxiety and depression scores ($P < .001$), and g) symptomatic medication use ($P < .001$) were significantly lower in the yoga group compared to the self-care group. The study was unequivocal about significant benefits from YI in migraine cases.

Improvement in Cardiac Autonomic Profile

A 2014 study showed that effectiveness of conventional therapy for migraines can be enhanced by making use of yoga techniques for neurological disorders. Improvements in vagal tone, reduced medical costs, lesser sympathetic activity have also been found in the same study.[47] This study was a clinical assessment of

YI in migraine management. The main objective of the study was to evaluate the efficacy of yoga as an adjuvant therapy for migraine. The methodology for the study was to assess clinical outcomes and conduct autonomic functions tests and explore if there was an improvement in quality of life (QOL) for migraine patients. There was random sorting of 30 patients into the conventional care group and 30 patients into the yoga intervention (YI) group. Besides conventional care the YI group received yoga practice session for five days a week over a 5-week timeline. There were two assessments for frequency of migraine episodes, intensity and the impact of headaches, first at the baseline period and the second time after the yoga training at the end of the timeline. The results given in Table 8 below show that both groups showed significant improvements in clinical variables, but the YI group had more conspicuous (note the three asterisks 'signifying very very significant') results in terms of more vagal tones and less reliance on sympathetic nervous system. Group Y numbers are comparatively more substantial like in the case of headache frequency and intensity. The vagal nerve is the tenth cranial nerve and is a critical component of the parasympathetic nervous system (PNS). The invocation and initiation of PNS is the raison d'etre of YI. PNS regulates body parts when the conscious mind is at rest. It showed that yoga therapy increased medical effectiveness of conventional treatment.

Table 8: YI in Migraine Headaches

Group	Pre	Post	Pre versus Post p-value
Headache frequency			
Group CC	10.5±3.8	5.2±2.1	<0.001***
Group Y	11.3±5.1	1.8±1.5	<0.001***
Group CC versus Group Y *P* Value	0.471	<0.001***	-
Headache Intensity			
Group CC	9.30±1.2	7.73±1.2	<0.001***
Group Y	8.70±1.3	2.03±1.3	<0.001***
Group CC versus Group Y *P* Value	0.059	<0.001***	-
HIT Score			
Group CC	75.4±0.9	68.6±4.6	<0.001***
Group Y	66.6±3.2	38.9±2.2	<0.001***
Group CC versus Group Y *P* Value	0.010*	<0.001***	-
HIT = Headache Impact Test; *P<0.05 Significant, **P<0.01 Very Significant, ***P<0.001 Very Very Significant			

Source: Kisan R. et al 2014, Y = Yoga Group, CC = Conventional Care Group

The study concluded that headache frequency and intensity were both reduced more in YI + conventional care group, than in the case of the conventional care group. There was cardiac autonomic balance improvement because of decrease in the drive of the sympathetic nervous system and also enhanced vagal tone.

A Migraine Case Study

A lady in her early forties, came to Temple Yoga with a serious, but not chronic case of throbbing headache diagnosed as migraine. The triggers in this case seemed to be changes in intensity of light and sound and also workplace anxieties because of a frenetic work pace. On a scale of ten (chronic pain) to zero (no pain) she averaged 6.5 over a month of recorded headaches. It would last a few hours some 9-10 days a month.

The condition was so disabling that while the patient understood the yoga techniques and how to perform them, she initially found it difficult to do even simple yoga exercises recommended as a cure: bhastrika or the bellows breathing exercise, ujjayi or the victorious breathing technique, viloma (alternate nostril breathing), pranayama (alternate nostril slow abdominal breathing), bhramari or exhaling and humming and sounding ZZHEE, like the humming bee. The ZZHEE sound has a vibrating feel over the face and frontal lobe of the head. Other exercises were Adhomukha Svanasana or the downward dog with or without props, and Sethubandasana or the bridge. This was followed by the corpse pose or the shavasana with a unique sequence of three phases. Under the influence of the exercises the cerebrospinal fluid begins to circulate more vigorously. The brain, ventricles, spinal cord and meninges feel stimulated. Thus the treatment improves oxygen nourishment to neurons and pacifies them, and eases stress.[48]

A self-evaluation by the patient after continuous practice for thirty days showed that the incidence of migraine was almost nil. Six months into migraine management convinced the patient that regular practice of this yoga drill is the best antidote to her migraine complaint both in chronic conditions after the headache has already started, and also as a prophylactic.

During the first two months there were five episodes of migraine of varying intensity according to the exercise log in a date-wise diary maintained by the patient. Despite continuance of the same work schedule she now felt that she had exited the "migraine tunnel." She was however cautioned to keep reassessing her work load and have "yoga breaks" whenever she could. Incidentally, in view of the difficulties of learning yogic techniques after the onset of problems such as migraine headaches, we recommend people learn them as a big stick to use against medical problems before they come. After much persuasion on our part and persistence on her side, regular daily morning practice of these exercises followed. This holistic approach involving mind and body for total wellness is the hallmark of treatments in yoga Chikitsa or treatment.

The overall conclusion this segment on migraines prompts is that YI is both effective as a cure and as a prophylactic. It is also cost-effective costing just a fraction of headache medication which may have other side effects, unlike YI. Today there is sufficient evidence[49] to support the claim that YI is holistic in improving physical and psychosocial health by means of, inter alia, down-regulating the hypothalamus-pituitary-adrenal axis as well as the SNS. At the same time it invokes the PNS with the help of GABA. Quality of life is enhanced and pain levels are reduced.

Prophylactics, Therapeutic Treatment and Robustness

So far we are looking at reducing health care costs by means of reducing illnesses in the first place and reducing the incidence of falling sick. But that is just one aspect of the use of yoga. Equally important, if not more, is the restoration of robust radiant health that yoga promises the practioner. The concomitant increase in productivity in every walk of life, improvement in the quality of decision-making, more innovations and patents, enhanced peace and harmony in the life of the people and the nation would elude attempts at quantification in dollar terms. The collateral advancements and upgrades in quality of life everywhere and in most citizens would be undreamed of. Yoga toughens the immune system. Now there is evidence that even in the case of congenital health issues, by boosting the lymphatic system together with spawning white blood cells in the bone marrow, energizing the spleen, thymus and complementary security components, yoga makes it easier to manage issues like Type I Diabetes, congenital heart weakness and similar inherited tricky health issues. The National Center for Alternative and Complementary Medicine has endorsed that yoga is mind-body medicine.[50]

- Yogic scientific techniques focus the mind on the work on hand by cutting out mental chatter.
- Yoga generates more alpha energy (bioelectricity) and takes the mind and body to the higher level of performance
- Yoga brings relaxation and internal awareness
- Yoga is energizing rather than fatiguing

Two effective techniques to cut down tension and stress are: Breathing and the Corpse pose. This is the urgent and rational need to include yoga as one of the mainstream therapies for tackling the persistent mental and physical ailments of humanity.

Most other modalities delve on the vegetative component of brain-body functions. They are somewhat oblivious of the internalized mind-body awareness. The awareness undertakes autopilot run of mind-body synchronization and harmonization. Patanjali school of yoga focused on psycho-somatic aspects of mind behavior or psyche function, and Swatmarama school concentrated on experiential relaxation during the transition from the somatic or body situation to the psychic plane. In one there is transition from the mind to the body, and in the second from the body to the mind in terms of synchronization and bringing both on line. The somatic and cortical awareness is handled by human information processing (HIP) pathway consisting of psychobiological 2-way 5-step processing, the two ways being conscious and unconscious, and the five steps being sensory inputs, cognition, short and long-term memory, conclusions and inferences, and executive use. This bio-apparatus regards yogic instruction as critical information. This is the primary biochemical mechanism that ushers in 'functional peace' after yoga exercise thanks to breath awareness. *(See Kulkarni DD, in Char S (2017), A compelling Call for Mix of Modality procedures at Chicago Meet, https://www.scivisionpub.com/pdfs/a-compelling-call-for-mix-of-modality-procedures-at-chicago-meet-269.pdf)*

Breath awareness triggers electro-cortical activity which in turn monitors and minimizes metabolic energy expenditure. This happens by means of modulation of psycho-neuro-immune (PNI) system via the neuroendocrine hypothalamic-pituitary axis. The scientific uniqueness of yoga is the enhanced signal power for cell-to-cell communications thus positively impacting both affective and cognitive homeostasis. Yogic HIP is more relaxing because of the two-step post-detection closure (PDC). HIP captures perceived somatic activity in both the detection and rejection stages. In the neural space it helps attain the neutral state of attention in the perceptual channel.

Kundalini Chakras - The Whirling Vortex of Quantum Level Energy

Clinical evidence about efficacy of yoga intervention (YI) is the focus of this book. There are not many scholarly papers about pressing into service Kundalini Chakras (KCs) as part of YI to address health issues. KCs have a role cut for them in realizing one's potentials and becoming more perfect and wonderful in the physical, mental and spiritual phases of life. It is a moot point whether basic *svastha* is a precondition for beginning to let the Kundalini Serpent uncoil itself. In view of this, KCs are included just in passing, more like an introduction. Also techniques such as breathing, meditation, lifestyle changes and others employed in KCs are familiar yoga procedures too. But Kundalini Yoga is not for the faint hearted.

Thus, there may not be an all-embracing case for KCs in this study. One cannot however, ignore the current interest in molecular level remedies for health issues such as cancer and heart disease, which has led to new explorations into the microcosm of Kundalini Chakras, each one a cognitive and extrasensory center. If yoga and meditation can help rouse the energy that lies coiled up like a cobra in the Muladhara Chakra down at the base site where the gender organs are located, it would help bring about much particle or molecular level remedies for contentious health issues.

Anyone willing to go through such an awakening is in for a radical change in one's lifestyle and in one's association with the world and its people. Such a person has to do a stark sankalpa to willingly go through such an experience and not want to go back to mundane existence. This fortitude is really an imperative and it is worth repeating that it is not for the weak-minded.Naturally there are not many takers. Riding that innate energy unleashed inside us, is like riding a bucking horse, only ten times more bucking. Many may be fated to fall off that high-energy horse, but some make it and they are venerated. It can only be speculated that the spiritual grand acharyas like Shankara, Ramanuja and Madhava were such realized persons as were several others: Meerabai, Ramana, Vallabh, Ramakrishna, Vivekananda, Chaitanya, Prabhupada, and many others. About the ascent of Kundalini in Jagadguru Sri Abhinava Vidyatheertha Mahaswamigal, Sringeri, see chapter 10 in Yoga, Enlightenment and Perfection, (2004), Sri Vidyateertha Foundation, Chennai.

To commence work on unleashing one's Kundalini seriously, is to pick up the gauntlet of evolution into a virtual super human being in this very life. One has to undergo a unique transformation and it could be mesmerizing. Rousing the Kundalini could cause chaos and havoc in the emotional domain of a person, but it would also help such a person to achieve one's full potential and become more godlike, along the lines of the meaning of "*Aham Brahmmosmi*" or "I am divinity." Besides superficial changes in food, clothing, personal appearance, livelihood, and relations with people including one's family members, by the time the Kundalini raises to the Sahasrara or the Pineal, or perhaps even before that, such a person is virtually reborn as someone else in terms of personality attributes. The genetic and other baggage of previous life seem to drop off. At one and the same time the person will feel a total disconnect with the near and dear, feel lonely like a space traveler (without communications with earthlings) and feel the real *vairagya* (total detachment) with life on terra firma. Terra firma itself need not be an illusion, but solid and firm. Accordingly, the same person in a vairagya mindset will, in terms of empathy, will feel your pain or ecstasy in endeavors and will reach out, be it a human being or even a creature.

CG Jung studied KC and his views rhyme with an expanding consciousness, the true intent of KC, albeit in a symbolic way. Jung, the Swiss psychiatrist, was one of the leading lights of analytical psychology and he applied his mind to deciphering the significance of the symbolism of KC to the duality the conscious and unconscious worlds.[51] Jung tried to understand KC through listening to his unconscious mind without a bias. Each Chakra had a particular symbolism. The inner messages from the unconscious mind, opposing a selected course of action, were to him the rational voice of nature or the unconscious (and the real) mind, "….. trying to correct an imbalance in consciousness."

Dreams, instincts, emotions, and some visions: Jung called for careful mapping of these experiences. Such mapping was done by Sri Abhinava Swamigal mentioned above, on his own, like others who have traversed the same path. Jung helped patients explore and individualize them and even helped patients understand their own psyche and the unfulfilled aspects of their personality. Such an effort, *a la* KC, would help the patient expand his/her consciousness and make such a person a fuller, if not a divine personality. We can postulate that every one may not be aspiring to reach the ultimate chakra of Sahasrara, but may settle for a much lower stage of evolution. Jung called this notional journey in (super) consciousness and its related narratives the archetypes of the collective unconscious.[52]

Once the Kundalini coil starts uncoiling there is a constant flow of energy. Unless one is used to riding a bucking horse, it is torturous riding on the unleashed vitality and momentum. The state of mind generated by a rising Kundalini is the ideal one for someone overwhelmed by any disease. It offers perhaps the best palliative care for such circumstances. Kundalini takes one into inner energy fields, in a more engineered manner than transcendental meditation which has more common place application. Kundalini is known to bestow supernormal abilities.

The sensations felt by one on the Kundalini path are different from chakra to chakra. By traditional reckoning there are seven chakras: Muladhara, Swadhinasthana, Manipura, Anahata, Vishuddhi, Ajna and Sahasrara through which one's soul is supposed to leave when it is time up for its host to go. Each Chakra or plexus, is the site of a key endocrine gland: the gonads (testes and ovaries) in the Muladhara periphery, adrenals in the Swadhisthana area, pancreas in the Manipura site, thymus in the Anahata Chakra, thyroid in the Ajna area, Pineal in the Vishuddha, and pituitary and hypothalamus in the Sahasrara as shown in Figure 7.

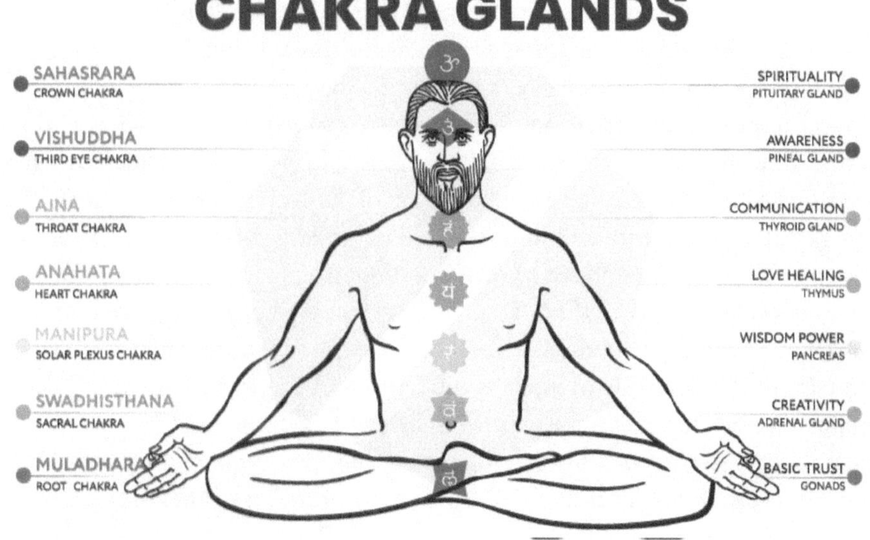

Fig 7: Chakra Glands

Source: Chakrastore.com

Each Chakra is also interconnected to three nadis: Ida on the left, Pingala on the right and Sushumna in the center of the spine. Ida associated with left nostril signifies the moon influence, Pingala, associated with the right nostril, the sun influence and Sushumna nadi is the trunk line for Kundalini vital energy to traverse from the Muladhara to the Sahasrara. Chakras and nadis are notional and psychic, and there is no structural or anatomical part that connotes them. By focusing on a given plexus when performing asanas, there is a good possibility of activating a body part or endocrine gland. For example when performing halasana if we shift the focus on to the Manipura chakra the pancreatic cells could function far better, generating all the needed insulin that helps keep the blood sugar at the optimum level.

According to those that have traversed this path, when Kundalini is passing through Muladhara chakra the sense of taste becomes acute, there is little fear of water, mental powers are enhanced, and for a while such a person may feel able to rein in one's destiny. Extra mundane perceptions become intense.

As Kundalini traverses through swadhinasthana the human gets clues such as heightened intuition, new sensations and perceptions. Further up as Kundalini enters Manipura there is loss of fat, there is radiance in face, reduced excretions and much less hunger. At the next higher up Anahata which is the site of the heart, the air one breathes becomes energetic prana. There is love for all mankind in a new kind of catholic mindset. As Kundalini enters the throat Chakra or the Vishuddhi Chakra there is a new resonance and tone to the voice which fascinates. Ajna Chakra dispels all ignorance and the person has much brilliance with wisdom. When Kundalini enters the final Sahasrara Chakra the person is considered perfect, like very divine. This is in fact a symbolization of the evolution of man both within one generation and within a human era. This is why each Chakra has a lotus flower which itself is symbolic of this evolution. The Sanskrit name of the lotus is *punkaja*, made up of *punka* or slush and *ja* meaning born. The lotus is born in slush, but by turning to the sun it blossoms out. The flower has a long stem which connects to the quagmire or slush at the bottom of the stem. Human life too is supposed to be drenched in quagmire out of which it is supposed to emerge. Like the lotus, it is supposed to blossom out in the sun, the sun signifying knowledge. Humans evolve into higher levels of conscience by turning to knowledge.

There are ways to press the Kundalini Chakras to work on the DNA. Yoga has the knowhow of dealing with transition areas between objective-subjective realms of this kind. It is wise to remember that much of the narrative about the Chakras is notional, not fully practical, but with guidance for adopting simple living and high thinking. As noted earlier there are no physical or substantiable body part like the Muladhara or the Sahasrara Chakras, but what it comes with are an aid to develop a) *vairagya* in the materialistic world and b) focus of hundred percent of one's energy on a singularity of merging the stream of consciousness within us with the macro or super-consciousness without. Further promoting this journey up are *bija mantras* for each Chakra, a geometrical *yantra*, separate for each Chakra, and a deity presiding within each Chakra and also a *vahana* or animal vehicle to move the energy.[53]

A skeptical mind will find it difficult to go along with the Kundalini system of energy getting impeded in the human body in the vortex of each chakra along the spine. As conscious energy starts its journey from the Muladhara to the Sahasrara it tries to overcome physical and psychic impediments including negative emotions such as anger, jealousy, disdain for cleanliness, depression, excessive indulgences, laziness and lethargy, tendency to go against the circadian flow and their like. In this effort the willpower of the individual is of utmost significance. Willpower should facilitate and smooth the flow of Kundalini energy all through the plexus, more like the surge of water, and unlike the gooey drift of lava.

Chapter 6

Yoga, Anxiety and Depression

Whenever there is any kind of threat it causes stress. Stress in turn generates anxiety. Threats could be real or perceived. Even if such fear is a product of hypochondria, it does not matter, it still causes stress and so anxiety. The physical offshoots of this nervousness of something bad or some harm, are eventually a) racing of heart which a person can feel, b) perspiring somewhat more than normal and c) also having perceptions of stress. Yoga has justifiably gained distinction as a leading remedy for stress and anxiety abatement. These woes are very much yoga's business, more so in the context of Surgeon General Vivek Murthy's book *Together* highlighting of the surge in drug overdose mortality due to the new loneliness caused by social distancing under COVID protocols.

One of the earliest studies, into mental disorders other than in India, was the Pilkington study (2005).[54] This looked into research during 1980s and early 2000. Those studies reported clinical outcomes of yoga intervention in psychic disorders including depression. The researchers reviewed several studies that came up on biomedical databases such as MEDLINE, EMBASE, CINAHAL, PsycINFO and the Cochrane Library, besides specialist complementary and alternative medicine (CAM) and the IndMED databases to identify unpublished, and ongoing research. The database search identified five randomized control trials. The yoga exercises used were however, different for the studies. And the severity of the mental illness condition was also varied, ranging from mild to severe.

While all five studies presented success in clinical outcomes, the British study found inadequacies in research protocols such as randomization methods, compliance and attrition rates. The study did not come across any adverse events due to yoga exercises other than fatigue and breathlessness in patients just in one of the studies. The British review of the five studies cautiously concluded that there were potentially beneficial effects of yoga intervention in depressive disorders. There must be further studies to particularize yoga treatment according to the severity of the disorder and the mobility of the patients, all of whom may not be able to do the exercises.

YI for Stroke Rehabilitation

One of the recent studies looked into the scope for use of YI for rehabilitation of victims of stroke in terms of recovery of function and quality of life (QoL). This study was undertaken by researchers in the department of nursing and community health in England.[55] Two RCTs (n = 72) that compared yoga with a waiting-list control or no intervention control were included in the study. The researchers concluded that in one study the effect of yoga on QoL spread over five domains viz., physical, emotion, communication, social participation, stroke recovery, was not significant. YI on memory domain was significant (mean difference (MD) 15.30, 95% confidence interval (CI) 1.29 to 29.31, P = 0.03). However the evidence for this finding was considered 'very low grade.' In the second study which used Stroke-Specific QoL Scale, no significant effect was found for YI. As far secondary outcomes such as movement, strength, endurance, pain and disability, as well as balance as measured by the Berg Balance Scale, the effect of YI was not significant (MD 2.38, 95% CI -1.41 to 6.17, P = 0.22). The effect was not significant for self-efficacy, gait, motor function, disability, anxiety, depression, and similar characteristics. However, a significant effect was found for anxiety: STAI-Y1 (MD -8.40, 95% CI -16.74 to -0.06, P = 0.05); the evidence for this finding was very low grade with high risk of bias. Large-scale investigations need to be undertaken to establish YI benefits for stroke rehabilitation. Perhaps it may also be prudent not to use 'very low grade' evidence, and use unbiased data so that the results are not vitiated and the conclusions may be relied upon. Research effort is also not wasted on data that may be contaminated.

PTSD in Women

Posttraumatic Stress Disorder (PTSD) in women is a particularly contentious mental issue and is likely to be more complex than in men. The hormones estrogen, progesterone and testosterone in both are the same, but there are differences in hormone production sites, blood concentrations, and hormone interactions with different organs, systems, and apparatus. For instance testosterone output in women is just 10 percent of that in men. Stress disorder is also more in the age group of 14-25 years. When it comes to release of hormones, the anterior pituitary does much the same for males and females. Beyond that however, for women it releases estrogen, a reproductive hormone for endometrial regrowth, ovulation and calcium absorption. Progesterone is the other biochemical that is secreted for inhibition of FSH (follicle stimulating hormone) and LH (luteinizing hormone) release.

It is believed that depression is more prevalent in young women than in men, one study stating that female: male ratio of global disability from major depression is 1.7: 1.0. The higher prevalence rate of depression among females is accounted for by variations in socioeconomic factors, including abuse, education and income.[56]

In a randomized controlled trial a 2014 study examined which symptoms of PTSD were reduced in response to YI. There were two groups to compare the effect of a YI with an assessment control.[57] The method employed by this study was examining if changes in psychological flexibility, mindfulness, and emotion regulation strategies (expressive suppression and reappraisal) were associated with posttreatment PTSD symptoms for 38 women with (Diagnostic and Statistical Manual of Mental Disorders, 4th Edition) full or subthreshold PTSD. Making use of hierarchical regressions, the study came up with interesting and surprising results too, like in (b and c): a) Compared to the control group, expressive suppression significantly decreased for the yoga group b) The control group surprisingly showed a significant increase in psychological flexibility, but not for the yoga group c) However, the unexpected outcome in (b) is possibly accounted for by the fact that increases in psychological flexibility were associated with decreases in PTSD symptoms for the yoga but not in the control group. The study concluded that by increasing psychological flexibility yoga may reduce expressive suppression and also improve PTSD symptoms.

Another study published in 2018 did a systematic study and meta-analyzed the effectiveness and safety of this modality to treat anxiety.[58] The researchers looked into all available randomized controlled trials (RCTs) that were done till October 2016 for the specific purpose of applying yoga for anxiety disorders and elevated levels of anxiety. The study set up four measurements: remission (reduction) rates in anxiety, depression, changes in quality of life and safety of the yoga techniques. The primary goal was anxiety level changes and the other three were secondary goals of the study. Included in the study were eight RCTs and the participants in the study numbered 319. The mean age (range) was given as 30.0 – 38.5 years.

The meta-analysis evidence for small short-term effects of yoga on anxiety compared to no treatment were as follows: standardized mean difference [SMD] = -0.43; 95% confidence interval [CI] = -0.74, -0.11; P =. 008), and large effects compared to active comparators, or those that receive similar but not same treatment, SMD = -0.86; 95% CI = -1.56, -0.15; P =. 02). Small effects on depression were found compared to no treatment: SMD = -0.35; 95% CI = -0.66,

-0.04; P =. 03. The effects were robust enough against potential methodological bias. The study could not find any effects in the case of persons whose anxiety disorders were measured by the Diagnostic and Statistical Manual criteria as well for others whose anxiety levels were measured by other criteria and for those with high elevated levels of anxiety.

A more recent 2019 study further underpins the findings of the above studies. There are some studies that compare the effects of traditional anti-depressants with YI in depression patients. The data show that YI comes out valuable in outcomes. YI does this by impacting neurotransmitters that regulate mood, motivation and pleasure.[59] The objective of the researchers was to evaluate effect of add-on yoga therapy on depression and comorbid anxiety. In this study patients with depressive disorder were allocated to either a standard antidepressant cum counseling group or to a YI group together with standard therapy. Montgomery–Asberg Depression Rating Scale and Hospital Anxiety and Depression Scale were used to rate depression and anxiety at baseline, 10th day and the 30th day. Only at baseline and the 30th day Clinical Global Impression (CGI) scale was applied to check on severity of illness and clinical improvement.

The results were that by the 30th day patients with YI had significantly lower scores of depression, anxiety and CGI scores as compared to the control group. Such a decline by way of a significant clinical improvement vis-à-vis the control patients was found for both the period between baseline and the 30th day as well as the period between the 10th to the 30th day. As far anxiety, the yoga group experienced significant decline in the baseline – 10th day period. The conclusion was that anxiety starts to decline by the 10th day even over short term YI and depression scores improve significantly over long term YI.

Which Yoga Modality for Depression?

Yoga exercises used in yoga intervention (YI) for depression are not the same and often been different. Also the asanas, breathing exercises, meditation and relaxation techniques have been used individually or in different combinations. So if these clinical studies are to be repeated, in what permutation/combination should they be used as a composite YI module? Such a module could be for a clinical trial or in the treatment of individual patients. Of particular interest was what specific outcomes can be expected from a matching of health complaints and yoga modules? These were the questions addressed in a study undertaken at the Department of Psychiatry, National Institute of Mental Health and Neuro Sciences, Bangalore.[60] The research objective was one of development and feasibility of yoga therapy module for out-patients with depression.

After a literature review, a program was developed matching yoga practices for clinical features of depression. The program thus developed consisted of Sukshma vyayama or subtle and loosening exercises, asanas, relaxation techniques, pranayama and chanting meditation. The duration of the treatment was two weeks. In order to validate the program after professional evaluation, a structured questionnaire was developed and submitted to nine experienced yoga professionals. The feedback was used to make changes in the program and was then tested on seven patients, five of them females, with the complaint of depression. The patients were recruited from the outpatient service of NIMH&NS, Bangalore.

One of the criteria for inclusion of a given exercise was it should receive a score of three or more on a 3-level scale that specified: moderately/very much/ extremely useful. Six out of nine experts suggested Sukshma Vyayama should be included. Five out of nine experts opined that 10 sessions (over 2 weeks) were inadequate to train the patients. All experts agreed that the module is easy to teach, learn and practice. Five patients who completed the module at the pilot stage expressed more than 80% satisfaction about the yoga practices and how they were taught. The main finding was that the severity of depression was substantially reduced both at 1 and 3 months follow-up. Thus it was concluded that the module developed by the research team at NIMH&NS and validated by experts in the field was both feasible and useful for treatment of depression.

YI for High-Risk Adolescents

This 2016 pilot randomized control trial was intended to test whether among high risk adolescents mindful YI was beneficial in cases of substance use and its psychological and psychophysiological correlates.[61] There have been evidence of positive effects on physical and emotional health. The study was conducted for students attending a school with high-risk of drop out. A 20-session YI was designed for this purpose. 50-minute classes were offered three times a week to students with a mean age of 16.7 years. In the yoga group there was a decrease in alcohol use as well as improved teacher-rated social skills (p < 0.10). The yoga group also showed a non-significant increase in arousal in response to relevant stimuli as measured in skin conductance. As regards hypothesized proximal measures of self-regulation, mood, mindfulness or involuntary engagement coping, there were no significant changes.

SNS, PSNS and GABA

Yoga's specialty in regard to anxiety, agitation, moods, depression, stress and so forth is the invoking and engagement of parasympathetic nervous system (PSN.) PSN is also known as vagal nerve. Yoga channels to PSN any stress from an event or trauma like disturbing distressing events in life such as accidents, disappointments, death, failures, mayhem, and trauma and their like. PSN works on the metabolism of the biochemical named thalamic gamma aminobutyric acid or GAMA. Its molecular formula is $C_4H_9NO_2$. GAMA is an inhibitory neurotransmitter in the central nervous system.[62] It functions as an inhibitory synapse and blocks adverse biochemical changes with the onset of bad news and events. Yoga helps GAMA levels to go up whereas anxieties, moods and stress lessen GAMA levels reducing the function of inhibitory GAMA. When yoga exercises and breathing are done by people with anxieties and major depressive disorders, GAMA levels in the system go up.

The evidence of increases in GAMA comes from several random control trials one of which is as recent as 2020.[63] In this PCT the intervention period was 12 weeks. As expected, symptoms of depression declined in the experimental group of persons with major depressive disorders or MDD. The experimental group was divided into a high dosage group with yoga intervention (YI) thrice a week, and a low dosage group receiving YI twice a week.

The group of psychiatrists and neurologists obtained baseline Thalamic GABA levels by means of using magnetic resonance spectroscopy at Scan-1 before randomization. After the assigned 12-week intervention, Scan-2 was obtained, immediately followed by a YI and Scan-3. Similarly Beck Depression Inventory II (BDI-II) scores were obtained before Scan-1 and Scan-3. All persons met the criteria for MDD. Ninety minute long Iyengar yoga exercises were done under each intervention. Breathing exercises, inter alia, consisted of doing five breaths per minute. The participants were asked to do yoga homework too. As a result of YI, there were significant improvements in BDI-ll levels. (Fig. 8) GABA levels significantly went up from Scan -1 to Scan 3, as well as from Scan 2 to Scan 3 in the LDG with a sample size of 15. There was a similar trend in the cohort group. Another important finding of this study was that the GABA levels remained high up to seven days after YI, but not after. The inference is that YI is needed at least once a week to keep GABA levels at higher levels, keep the metabolism of GABA at a healthy level and otherwise constantly benefit from improved moods and otherwise fight depression.

GABA Levels

Several studies of a similar nature have been done before this study and they underscore the same findings as regards YI impact on MDD and worse. More serious question of suicidal ideation (SI) has been addressed with yoga intervention and with encouraging results. One such 2018 RCT study looked into the effects of Iyengar YI together with yogic breathing for persons with MDD as well as with SI without intent.[64] YI was for a period of 12 weeks as in the 2020 study. Each class was for a duration of 90 minutes. There were 30-minute homework sessions too.

The criteria for admission into the study was that the participant should have a BDI score of greater than or equal to 14. 32 persons were randomized into low dose group (LDG) with two classes or HIGH Dose Group (HDG) with three classes per week. 30 persons completed the protocol. At initial screening 9 participants validated SI without intent. After YI, eight out of these 9 persons reported resolution of SI. Musculoskeletal pain was associated in 15 out of 17 adverse reporting. Such pain was resolved over the course of the study. Thus YI may reduce SI without intent and could also resolve issues related to MDD.

GABA levels get reduced when a person has mood and anxiety disorders. As a matter of fact, pharmacologic formulations are prescribed to increase GABA levels to improve moods. Some of such formulations are nitric oxide synthase inhibitors, cannabinoid agonists (CB1 receptor agonists), cholecystokinin receptor 1 (CCK1) antagonists, and others. When GABA levels go down there is also a reduction in the inhibition of neurotransmission in the central nervous system. With that, the conscious mind in the cortex is more exposed to the deleterious impact of bad news or damaging activity. Wear and tear caused by continuous exposure to stress - the fight or flight ecosystem – increases.

Yoga helps rise the GABA levels and thereby helps as a synaptic inhibitor and curbs neurotransmission, and decreases aggravation of anxieties and fears. Positive correlations have been found between improved mood and decreased anxiety and thalamic GABA levels. Thus inner biochemical and endocrine balance is restored and a modicum of peace is refurbished. The human mind remains unperturbed and no wear and tear due to stress occurs. Yogic activity thrusts GABA level up and restores calm and peace.

There were questions whether any physical activity besides yoga can have the same impact on enhancing GABA levels in the mind or whether it was specific to yogic activity. To test this out, a clinical trial was undertaken 2010.[65] Subjects with no significant medical or psychiatric disorders were randomized to yoga exercises or to a metabolically matched walking exercise to last 60 minutes, 3 times a week for 12 weeks. The researchers recorded the mood and anxiety scales at weeks 0,4,8,12, before a magnetic resonance spectroscopy scan. There was a baseline Scan 1 and another, Scan 2, at the end of the 12 weeks. Soon after this second scan there was a 60-minute yoga session or a walking intervention, to be followed by Scan 3. The results were that the 19 subjects in the Yoga group experienced greater improvement in moods and decline in anxiety than the walking group with 15 subjects. Greater improvement in mood and bigger decreases in anxiety were reported in the yoga group than in the walking group.

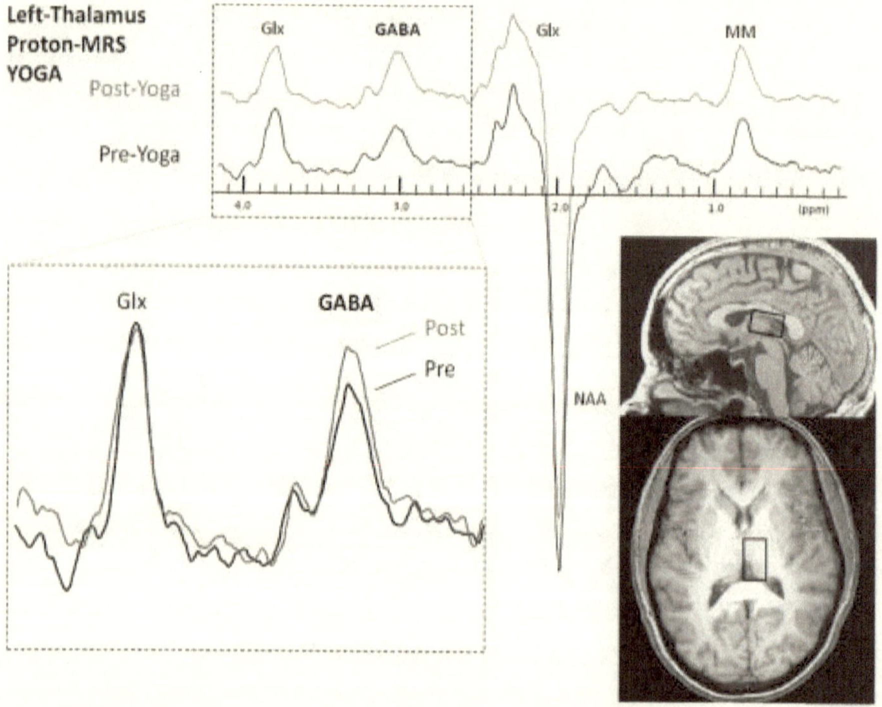

Fig. 8: Yoga Boosts GABA

Source: Streeter CC et al 2010

Autonomous and Parasympathetic NS

It has already been observed above that the autonomous nervous system consists of both the sympathetic and parasympathetic nervous systems: SNS and PSNS. When stress takes over a person, or when a person feels threatened, SNS goes on overdrive and initiates more than 1400 biochemical processes linked to the mind, body, emotions and behavior for safeguarding survival. There are bodily changes in an emergency, like vasoconstriction or narrowing of blood vessels, increased blood pressure and heart rate, shortness of breath and allied signs. The lever begins to convert glycogen into glucose. Less blood flows to the extremities and to the digestive system. There is some bronchial dilation. By now, or even much earlier, the hypothalamus-pituitary-adrenal axis would have been activated. The hypothalamus releases CRF: corticosteroid releasing factor and the pituitary releases ACTH: adrenocorticotropic hormone and the adrenal glands release cortisol. Cortisol has a useful function of metabolizing fat, protein, and carbohydrates. Glucose gets converted into gluconeogenesis.

The problem is that over a longer term, depending upon the coping capability of a person, excessive stress will have deleterious effect of suppressing the immune system, increasing retention of sodium and water in the kidney, increased blood volume and blood pressure, and also higher blood concentration. At this stage, there is negative feedback to cut down release of ACTH from pituitary and CRF from the hypothalamus. Homeostasis starts happening and body parts start coming back to normalcy, coming back on track. But if the body continues to experience stress over real or perceived threats, the HPA axis is activated again. There is more release of biochemical hormone - epinephrine or adrenalin which serves as a neurotransmitter. And the cycle starts afresh. Frequent HPA activation will start numerous health issues that concern the mind, the heart, the digestive system, immune system, and soon cancer too will start flaunting its ulcers, cysts, lumps, tumors and leukemia.

Yoga comes to the rescue. Yogic asanas and breathing, besides the yogic perspective, invoke the parasympathetic nervous system (PSNS). PSNS is activated when there is yogic relaxation. PSNS reduces the cortisol hormone and reduces the damage due to stress via the HPA axis activation. As we saw earlier, yoga boosts GABA: Gamma aminobutyric acid which somewhat inhibits neuron networking. This causes less reaction to emotions in the limbic system and more on the left side: the left frontal cortex. There is a medical or pharmacological way of bringing this about with mood medications and antidepressants (SSRIs) and antianxiety drugs. There may be side effects and may also be addictive. There is hardly an alternative to yoga exercises as a routine activity and better still, as a way of life, thereby managing stress like a champ. Only at serious peril to our physical and mental health can we afford to forget that stress is the root cause of 85 percent or more of all health problems.

Stress is what drives much of this world and its activities. Nevertheless, excessive stress, beyond one's capability to cope with it, causes a surfeit of inflammation which impedes immune activity by decreasing the number of immune cells, increases susceptibility to cancer, enlarges the amygdala, decreases GABA, impairs memory, lessens cognitive ability, reduces metabolic activity, quickens aging and causes many related negative developments.

Chapter 7

Yoga and Immune System

It would be a *faux pas* to omit what yoga does to the Immune System, the body's internal security system. The lymph nodes occur all over the body. They are incredibly sophisticated, and as a critical component they respond reliably and consistently to yoga practices. The immune cells are all the time fighting invading virus, bacteria, fungi, parasites (VBFP) other pathogens that cause disease. This vital part of our body, the first line of defense against VBFP consists of white blood cells, spawned in the spongy tissues of the bone marrow, the lymphatic nodes, the thymus, the spleen and other complementary units including the skin, the digestive track, and the cilia. Besides the lymph nodes, the tonsils, the appendix, adenoids and even the intestines have T cells which like the lymph nodes clean up germs and dead cells. While the circulatory system has the heart to pump blood all over the body, the lymph liquid has no pump and it circulates on its own and of course it is body movement that aids it the most. And the movements need not be as strenuous as jogging, but just simple ones likes yanking gently the ear lobes, fast-breathing Bhastrika or Kapalabhati, and heal-toe exercises. About two liters of colorless fluid circulate all over the body through lymphatic ducts, tubes, vessels, nodes and tissues. The lymph nodes have blood vessels from which the nodes absorb water and proteins among others. There is much functional link between the blood venous system and the vascular system in lymph nodes.[66]

White blood cells (WBC) or lymphocytes are the watchdogs looking for alien materials injurious to humans like VBFP and other toxic stuff identified in the antigens on top of invading microbes. WBC include B-cells or B-lymphocytes that secrete antibodies. WBC also have T-cells and killer cells, each one with a designated function. For example, T-cells go after virus and cancer cells, whereas B-cells go after bacteria. Killer cells pack off invading microbes.

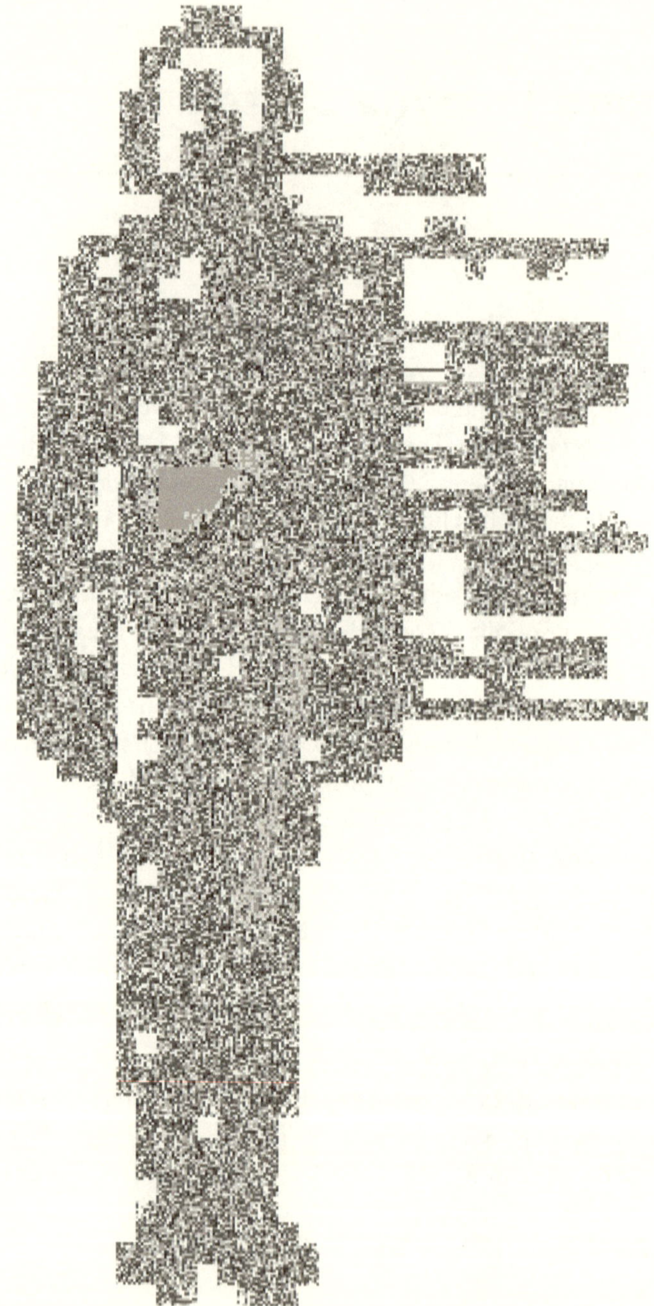

Fig 9: The Immune Defense

Source: www.lgdalliance.org/the-lymphatic-system

The lymphatic structure is made up of a) lymph nodes or glands that capture illness-causing microorganisms, b) vessels, ducts and tubes that carry the lymph liquid all over the body c) the blood-filtering spleen and others. The lymph liquid is the medium for WBC to move all over the human body, and capture microorganisms (visible on microscopes that magnify them tens of thousands of times.) Lymph nodes are there in the neck, in the groin and behind the knee (the red dots in Fig. 9.)

Besides filtering blood, the spleen also recycles old red blood cells. Spleen fights certain kinds of bacteria that cause meningitis or pneumonia. Yet another key task performed by the spleen is the making of antibodies and lymphocytes. Antibodies single out invading microbes by recognizing the antigens on the microbes. Once such microbes are marked harmful they are done away with. There are other microorganisms that are allowed to stay and multiply.

One of the essential parts of the immune system is the thymus located behind the sternum in the chest. The hormone thymosin promotes production of T-cells needed for fighting virus. But it stops growing by the time body reaches puberty and starts to shrink into a fatty tissue. But luckily by puberty it would have produced all the T-cells needed for a lifetime. Cilia is a hair-like contraption that helps mucus in the lungs to be brushed up, so it could be coughed out by the throat.

Yoga Ensures Lymph Health

Yoga massages the immune and endocrine system and some of the asanas serve the same purpose that the heart does for blood circulation: the exercises help pump the colorless lymph liquid throughout the body through lymph glands, vessels, tubes and so forth. Fast-breathing exercises like Bhastrika and Kapalabhati stimulate the flow of lymph liquid (or plasma) by mobilizing the thoracic area. Asanas that activate the lymph system are the padmasana (lotus), vajrasana or sitting with the calf muscle pressed, utkatasana or the chair posture, Garudasana or the wrapping of one leg over the other in a standing position, the bridge pose, and many others that squeeze the calf muscle and the stomach, or help turn the neck, pelvic region, arms, mooladhara (inguinal) area and others, that are the location of lymph nodes. Asanas that impact the clavicular bones improve the flow in the lymph drainage. Bhastrika and such other breathing act on the diaphragm below the chest with the same effect.

One of the common finishing asanas in Temple Yoga class is the torso twist in prone position without lifting the shoulder blades, and placing the knees one upon on the other. Yoga works on the joints where the lymph nodes are strategically located by altering the pressures, thereby activating them and improving the flow of the lymph fluid. Yoga also lets the parasympathetic nervous system take over and cuts the amount of stress the sympathetic nervous system handles by letting the parasympathetic nervous system handle stress. This cutback of stress on the sympathetic system is a major boost for improving the health of the immune system.

Other easy ways to improve the flow of lymph is drinking more water, deep abdominal breathing, hot and cold showers, not wearing tight clothes, and consuming saatvic food.

A 2011 study about the impact of yoga on stress levels of MBBS medical students during examination time showed that the control group that did not undergo any yoga training suffered much more stress compared to the experimental group that had yoga training for 35 minutes every day for 12 weeks. Besides the impact on the immune system of future physicians during their examination time, the study also looked into physiological parameters such as blood pressure, heart rate, respiratory rate, and psychological parameters. Also assessed were Global Assessment of Recent Stress Scale and Spielbergers State Anxiety score at baseline and during the examination. Serum cortisol levels, IL-4, and IFN-γ levels were determined by enzyme-linked immunosorbent assay technique.

There were significant changes in the control group in physiological parameters during examination time, as well as in psychological indicators like stress. The study showed *highly significant difference* in control group compared with *significant difference* in yoga group. During the examination, the increase in serum cortisol and decrease in serum IFN-γ in the yoga group was less significant ($P<0.01$) than in the control group ($P<0.001$). Increase in serum cortisol indicates some tension and decrease in interferon gamma (IFN-γ) signifies reduced immune response. Both the groups demonstrated an increase in serum IL-4 levels, the changes being insignificant for the duration of the study. In the light of these results, the study concluded that Yoga fights autonomic changes and damage of cellular immunity seen in examination stress.[67]

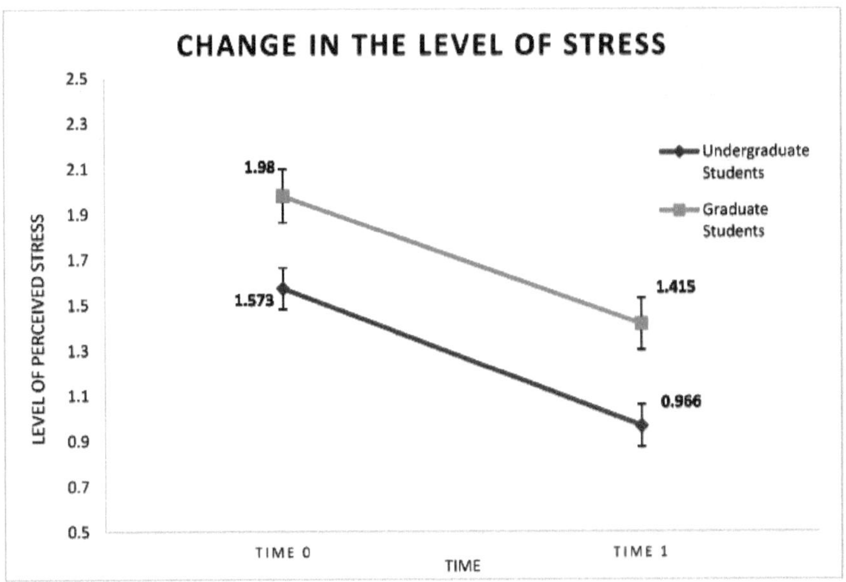

Fig. 10: Stress Level Changes

Source: Cozzolino M et al 2020

Similar to the MBIs is the Mind-Body transformation therapy (MBT-T) previously known as creative psychosocial genomic healing experience © (CPGHE).[68] Two sets of students participated in the study: first year university students and post-graduate students in psychotherapy. All 159 students were given a single session of MBT-T in two separate sessions. Paired sample t-tests showed that there was a statistically significant reduction in stress between pre- and post-intervention states in both the samples (t_{88} = 5.39, p < 0.001; t_{53} = 4.56, p < 0.001 respectively). The intervention showed that regardless of the perceived level of stress and also the educational level, MBT-T helped reduce stress in both first year university students as well as in post graduate students with expertise in the domain of well-being.

The autonomic nervous system serves as a bridge or communication link between the brain and the immune system. Yoga helps the endocrine system, and keeps the hypothalamus particular in high spirits. It signals the immune mechanism to be on a high healthy alert to take on onslaughts from virus and bacteria. Many more studies of this kind to highlight the security protection offered by yoga exercises against stress-caused cell debility are available. A comprehensive 360° view of autonomic-immune physiological dispensation is available in the Kenney-Ganta study.[69] Thus by reining in stress, yoga is able to strengthen the body's defense mechanism and enable it to be more of a deterrent against virus, bacteria, fungus and their like.

Chapter 8

Common Sense, Cognition and Judgement in Decision-making

The question that pops up in the mind of the yoga practioner who watches other people suffer illnesses is: Is that suffering inevitable or unavoidable? It is sad that there is so much suffering due to poor health caused not as much by congenital or infectious disease, which are explicable, but more on account of life styles which may not be conducive to harboring vigorous health. Many of us take good health for granted. Daily Activities of Life (DAL) or Activities of Daily Life (ADL) relate to numerous decisions we take in a routine manner, generally on the basis of customs and practices, folkways and mores, traditions or superstitions and habits. Some decisions are impulsive, and not taken after some cool thinking about the pros and cons of the decision. More often many decisions are of this kind when some folks go shopping The choices people make about dividing time between various activities more often than not, border on squandering the limited time we have, often so rash as to bring trouble and ill health.

The ADL decisions often relate to when to wake up, what chores to do first, whether you should go through media messages on Twitter, Face Book, WhatsApp or go brush teeth and wash face, warm up and do exercises (what type of exercise or go walk, walk on the terrace or at the Park?), whether to drink coffee or tea, how strong a coffee, with milk/sugar or without, when to bathe, eat breakfast, what kind of breakfast and lunch to eat, veg or non-veg, and hundreds of decisions of this kind besides numerous official chores for which we get paid. These official chores too offer choices though to a very limited extent unless you are someone like Elan Musk, Bill Gates, Jeff Bezos, or Mark Zuckerberg. Also critical is what mindset we have vis-à-vis people we meet, regardless of frequency, and how we deal with them, how much we laugh in a day, how much water we drink to keep ourselves well-hydrated and also how much are we learning? There is an endless number of choices and decisions to make, some very consequential like the choice of a life partner or career education, and some not so consequential, like whether to drink milk or have coffee. Not infrequently, choices are made unthinkingly!

When persons in authority like the parents or the Headmaster of the School or the Minister (Secretary) of education, or leaders of the country make decisions uncaringly for the rest of us, there is far-reaching turmoil and even disaster. What follow are simple but convincing examples of common sense solutions to curb illness and costs. These solutions gain much significance for about 28 million Americans who 'manage' their health care without health insurance and also for those with more than adequate health insurance, but whose escalating health care costs bring them close to financial collapse. In India the Ayushman Bharat Pradhan Mantri Jan Yojana (AP-PMJAY) hopefully would engage more indigenous modalities for the cure of illnesses. That would enable coverage of more people in a universal health care system.

Laughing as Medicine

Most of the time, it is interactions with people that perturb us and cause stress. The real need to laugh and maintain good cheer cannot be taken too lightly. The Epilogue chapter at the end of the YVM deals with it in more detail. Laughing is one of the best remedies for various problems. It clears stale air and harmful thoughts inside and anchors the mind on the right attitude to problematic people and contentious problems. The Help Guide[70] lists the following physiological benefits of laughter: boosts immunity, lowers stress hormones, decreases pain, relaxes your muscles and prevents heart disease. The mental health benefits listed are: adds joy and zest to life, eases anxiety and tension, relieves stress, improves mood and strengthens resilience. The following social benefits of laughter are also listed in the same website: strengthens relationships, attracts others to us, enhances teamwork, defuses conflict, and promotes group bonding.

Critical Thinking on Key Questions

More critical thinking goes into questions with a decisive influence on quality of life, such as what academic qualifications to acquire, what courses to take, who to work for, where to live, whom to marry, whom to befriend, whether to adopt family planning as regards progeny or let nature have its way, how much to provide for the rainy day, for retirement, for children's (grandchildren's) education, and scores of such questions, most of which are interrelated.

At times the health and wellness angle is ignored such as when we decide about taking on extra assignments or business contracts because it is taken for granted that whatever decisions are taken are all safe and appropriate to one's station, global outlook, career, age, and so forth. Some of the consequences of bad decisions are headaches/health issues directly as a result of binging the previous night, stomach upsets because of bad/inappropriate food, losses and injuries due to unthinking acts of even family members and friends, and most commonly, whiling away time entertaining oneself, or absurdly indulging in something absolutely unconnected to immediate duties and goals of life (if any!), dharmas or pressing tasks with deadlines. The penchant to indulge in irrelevancies of life, instead of focusing on immediate and long term goals, is universal. Even for those contemplating their pointlessness in life, tough health is essential.

Common Sense about Food Consumption

One of the most common indulgences relates to overeating or indulging or not paying attention to calories consumed. Overweight and what is worse, obesity are the result of such indulgence. And obesity is the mother of most diseases. Also it is not rocket science to learn how to hold weight down to fitness levels. One could, for a start, begin minimizing if not cutting out high-calorie foods: sugar, carbs and fat, and committing oneself to regular walking, exercise or yoga. Regularity is of utmost importance. Yoga exercises can be done at home with minimum or no equipment and in all weathers. Second, there is intermittent fasting. A 2018 study in the form of a meta-analysis of four studies covering the period of 2000 – 2018, found that intermittent fasting leads to significant decrease in fat mass (P-value <0.01.) Equally heartening was the conclusion that such fasting resulted in the reduction in low-density lipoprotein and triglyceride. (P-value < 0.05.) This study unequivocally concluded that intermittent fasting was efficient in reducing weight, regardless of BMI.[71]

Most of us know that 'an ounce of prevention is better than a pound of cure' but not many care to practice this principle until it is too late. Both in India and in America more and more people are becoming **overweight,** body-mass-index or BMI going above 25, or even **obese** with BMI exceeding 30. Incidentally you calculate BMI by multiplying your body weight in pounds by a multiplier of 703, and then divide this product by your height in inches². (Alternatively you can visit http://www.nhlbisupport.com/bmi/ and get a computation of your BMI.) The simple formula is:

*BMI = (WEIGHT in pounds) * 703) / HEIGHT ² in inches*

Overweight and obese persons, whose numbers are going up in America, increase the risk for many diseases and health conditions. Healthline website data provides useful information.[72] 36.5 percent of American adults are obese and another 32.5 percent of American adults are overweight. This means 69 percent or over two-thirds of American adults are overweight or even worse. One in six children in the US is obese. Some sixty chronic diseases are linked to obesity. Particular mention may be made of arthritis, asthma, diabetes, heart disease, stroke, cancer, and many others. Not surprisingly overweight/obese persons spend more per capita, $1429 on health care than others, or a total of $147 billion. While more males are overweight than females, more females (40.4%) are obese than males (35%). Children who are obese tend to be overweight or obese as adults too. Ethnicity also is a factor with obesity. 48.4% of African-Americans, 42.6% of Hispanics, 36.4% Caucasians and 12.6% of Asian Americans are obese.[73]

Virtues of Fasting

Not very different from intermittent fasting, is the means to obtain nutrients for purposes of overall fitness and reducing the risk of overweight and obesity. The widely-acccepted answer is an adherence to vegetarian diet. It is now widely accepted that vegetarian diets are far better in terms of providing needed calories, and far better than other non-plant foods. The Physicians Committee for Responsible Medicine (PCRM) reviewed the evidence about plant-based foods, and only thereafter underlined the health benefits of such a diet. It is higher in fiber and lower in cholesterol and fat compared to omnivorous diet, leave alone carnivorous diets, besides scoring higher on the Healthy Eating Index (HEI). The PCRM took the opportunity to also include other major advantages of plant-based diet: a) Protection against type 2 diabetes b) Reduced risk of heart disease and cardiometabolic-related deaths.[74]

Lesson from COVID-19: Cut Non-Veg Food

Not surprisingly there is an increasing trend towards plant-based diets. In America, the percent of vegan diet consumers has gone up from 1% in 2014 to 6% in 2017. In this discussion what is not lost is the fact that the preference for plant diet is also on account of compassion for all living creatures. Man has come a long way from the hunter-gatherer carnivore period and even from omnivore times, to pure vegetarian days. Of course, there are communities caught up in each one those epochs as well as in the transition phases.

In a civilized society there does not seem to be much place for slaughter houses or manipulation of the animal biochemistry to make them yield more of anything, like for example, milk. Not the least important, more resources are needed to bring up the supply chains for meat. Overeating and bingeing and even sheer waste are also common place where such indulgences are afforded. A study by Pimental & Pimental published as early as in 2003 had noted that the daily quantity of calories consumed was as high as 3533 kcal per person as against the RDA norm of just around 2000 calories, depending upon active or sedentary disposition or occupation, gender and age group. The number of persons depending on a plant-based diet worldwide is about 4 billion which is double the number of persons living on a meat-based diet. The food industry in America consumes 80% of fresh water, occupies 50% of the land area and burns up 17% of fossil energy used in America. The study also concluded that in terms of environmental sustainability, the meat-based food system requires more energy, land and water resources than the lacto-vegetarian diet, because of which the latter is more sustainable.[75]

One of the nonpharmacological means to reduce blood pressure is vegetarian diet. Hypertension can be easily reduced and managed by diet. One of the studies supporting such conclusion is by Yokoyama et al (cited below.) This study reviewed evidence from seven clinical trials and 32 observational. The data was extracted from articles in Medline and Web of Science between 1946 -2013 and from 1900 to 2013 respectively. This was a meta-analysis of studies examining the associations between vegetarian diets and BP. Vegetarian diets generally exclude meats and some may include dairy, eggs and fish. Otherwise such diets are plant-based and include mainly vegetables, grains, nuts, legumes and fruits.

Superiority of Veg Diet for BP

The results of the meta-study were as follows: In the 7 controlled trials (a total of 311 participants; mean age, 44.5 years), consumption of vegetarian diets was associated with a reduction in mean systolic BP (-4.8 mm Hg; 95% CI, -6.6 to $--3.1$; $P<.001$; $I^2=0$; $P=.45$ for heterogeneity) and diastolic BP (-2.2 mm Hg; 95% CI, -3.5 to 1.0; $P<.001$; $I^2=0$; $P=.43$ for heterogeneity) compared with the consumption of omnivorous diets. In the 32 observational studies (a total of 21 604 participants; mean age 46.6 years), consumption of vegetarian diets was associated with lower mean systolic BP (-6.9 mm Hg; 95% CI, -9.1 to -4.7; $P<.001$; $I^2=91.4$; $P<.001$ for heterogeneity) and diastolic BP (-4.7 mm Hg; 95% CI, -6.3 to -3.1; $P<.001$; $I^2=92.6$; $P<.001$ for heterogeneity) compared with the consumption of omnivorous diets. Vegetarian diets are thus a proven nonpharmacological means of reduction of BP.[76]

Over-Testing the Obvious?

If and when sickness occurs, the immediate reaction in many a people innocent about the pathology and physiology of a human system, is to panic and agree to the medical system's over-testing, over-treatment and over-medication. Hospitals in USA have charged $500 for a blood test, $5000 for three stitches in an emergency room, $50,000 for minor outpatient foot surgery and $500,000 for three days in a hospital after a heart attack. The payments for inflated bills are often wheedled out under threat of collection.[77] Prof. Atul Gawande, MD, compared the Medicare costs per annum per enrollee in two neighboring cities of McAllen and El Paso, Texas, and found that in 2006 El Paso where the enrollees were somewhat healthier had almost exactly one half the cost of McAllen: $7504 in El Paso and $15,000 in McAllen. The doctors were ordering needless tests in McAllen. Some physicians had investments in the firms that owned testing facilities. One of the senior doctors there admitted to Gawande that the main stimulus for a doctor earlier was "… how to do a good job. Now it is about how much will you benefit?"[78]

Among the lay public, it is never the case to get to know the health issue, whether it is a simple cold or a life-threatening cancerous growth, to get a better grasp of the problem. Over the counter drugs, so freely available are used indiscriminately even when nonpharmacological (grandma) remedies are available. Dazzling publicity for pharma drugs for even minor ailments like colds, coughs and fever are ubiquitous and crowd out remedies regarded by misinformed persons as fuddy-duddy such as different kashayams (herbal concoctions together with hot spices), turmeric powder, hot water, thin coating of scented Vaseline on the inner walls of the nostrils for allergic colds and sneezes, gurgling with hot salt water for throat irritation and coughs, and scores alike. May be it is not a bad idea to conduct RCTs for gurgling with hot salt water for throat irritation and present the results in JAMA or Lancet for wider acceptance of the grandma prescription?

Diaphragmatic or Belly Breathing

Speaking of common sense in health care, most people don't even breathe right, indulging in short and shallow breaths, paradoxical breathing and not knowing deep abdominal breath. Neurosurgeon the late Paul Kalanithi in his book 'When Breath Becomes Air', quotes Baron Brooke Fulke Greville's poem:

You that seek what life is in death

Now find it air that once was breath.

In Sanskrit language breath is prana or life force which Baron Greville's words above are calling attention to. Otherwise it is just lifeless air. The critical significance of breath is lost on most persons. This conclusion is based on how many persons seldom have deep abdominal breath as the default pattern. Deep breath in quantitative terms such as milliliters per breath is discussed under the 'Yoga and Asthma' chapter.

Yogic Breathing with Omkara

The benefit in yogic breathing even while chanting the Omkara mantra in step and style with inhalation, holding and exhalation is that one attains serenity and silence. The meaning of AUM: Srushti, sthithi and laya or creation, preservation and recycling respectively are represented by A, U and M. When it is chanted synchronously with deep abdominal breathing musing over the three facets of the universe, there is a unique sense of oneness with the Creator or with innate intelligence, followed by complete serenity and silence. This experience resonates with toughening and supporting the immune cells.

Ayurveda and yoga provide affordability, accessibility as well as applicability, they being so indigenous and most Ayurvedic drugs being of high quality too. But the fact remains that the rest of the population suffers from life-limiting diseases. A health care system fully integrated with Yoga-Ayurveda and indigenous systems can attend to this massive health care challenge.

Offered above are simple-sounding and common sense solutions that are often taken for granted and otherwise neglected or belittled as in the case of as elementary an essential function as deep breathing. As a matter of fact, such neglect of common sense chores run into hundreds. One glaring neglect of that kind is not wearing masks or not maintaining distance between people even in these COVID-19 times. Consequently there are immediate spikes in COVID cases wherever the protocols are not adhered to. The common sense instances given above of overeating, not adhering to healthy habits such as exercising and walking, indulging in entertaining oneself till one 'drops dead' on account of fatigue and many more, are but issues of life style choices. They sound rather too simple and elementary, but do have life altering outcomes. There are also societal or nationwide benefits too in terms of savings of hard tax dollars or people's tax contributions in health care costs as discussed in Chapter 3.

Chapter 9

Yoga and the Genes

The human cell is a microcosm of the human body which in turn is a microcosm of the universe made up of the same cosmic or star dust of Big Bang. The human body is a hologram of the universe which resonates with what the ancient and ageless Vedas taught a very long time ago: *Yatha Brahmande, Thatha Pindande.* This translates roughly to: as is the primal cosmos, so is the microcosmic embryonic body. Everything in the universe, the elements in particular, all 118 of them you find in the Periodic Table of Chemical Elements, are in the human body. This reminds one of quantum physics of subatomic particles overlapping into the unified field theory that occupied Albert Einstein almost in the 11th hour of his life.

Yogic science attained a modicum of success in capturing the deep truths in the patterns that become apparent at the micro and macrocosm levels. Yoga's treatment modus operandi is also well informed of this deep connection, enabling its holistic ways in dealing with health issues, as part of its exploration of pathogenesis, or the roots of disease.

The idea of inheriting characteristics from previous generations has been with mankind for long. Thus we say: As is the father, so is the son. Eugenics, a word coined in 1883 by Francis Galton was all about selective breeding of humans so that the very best of humans with the best of health, intelligence and with maximum competence would populate the world. Such an advanced population would not have any violence in thought, word and indeed, perhaps? Eugenics would populate the land without any of the shortcomings or physical or mental weaknesses. Eugenics however leads to preventing groups with deficiencies in good looks, education, character and other features from having offspring that would be a burden to society. Sterilization of women in those communities was talked of. Instead eugenics encouraged family planning.

In India amongst Hindus, *sa-gothra* or close cousin marriages within the same lineage (*gothra*) were frowned upon for the reason of making it hard to inbreed. Behind all that critiquing of cousin marriages was the desire for fresh blood that would help come up with better versions of humans or improve the human race. The entire discussion became a great divider of people with weaker sections protesting that it would all go downhill into racist plot against colored people. Also who was to decide who is better as a human being? And how would it not be a subjective and selective breeding of a superior class?

GENE ENVIRONMENT AND *PRANAMAYA KOSHA*

Genes, which according to the Human Genome Project number about 20,000 to 25,000 in the human body, are the latest buzz words, but yoga jargon such as *anna maya kosha* and *prana maya kosha* take account of genes too in their anatomical and physiological span. *Prana* or the life energy force of breathing oxygen-rich air pervades the entire body by means of being there in the cells and neurons. *Prana* is a *sine quo non* for generating energy through the process of oxidative phosphorylation. The gene environment, if not the gene *per se*, is still very much within the sphere of human tweaking. To that extent yoga helps manage gene typos and mutations, the phenotype, even if not the genotype.

It is possible that the influence of genetics is strong and some genetic mutations trigger instant changes without preceding symptoms and red signals of any kind. There is the case of the mother of Sonia Vallabh. Her mother, otherwise healthy, suddenly developed dementia, wasted away and died apparently for no reason (also see page 89 about prion). Ms. Sonia is supposed to have inherited this defective gene and is seeking a shield of a prophylactic for preventing the same kind of dementia that may be a potential life hazard for her. Charles Mayo MD, founder of Mayo Clinic in1924 said: That which can be foreseen can be prevented. If for instance, we know that obesity, if not overweight, is a significant factor in numerous illnesses including cardiac diseases, cancer, diabetes, backache, and a host of others, should we not prevent it from occurring in the first place? Much of the human race is so intensely immersed in the chores or activities of daily life (ADL) that they are either apathetic and indifferent, or ignorant of the means to better physical or mental fitness. It is not yet known if Sonia Vallabh found a prophylactic shield against her inherited hazard. Perhaps she should be researching into Ayurveda and Yoga for a better answer.

Intensive immersion into yoga may offer such a shield or vaccination against common ailments. However, in a different contextual setting there is no cure against cognitive dissonance, knowing for example that gene phenotype can be influenced for the better through yoga modality and still ignoring yoga.

YOGA AND GENE UP- OR DOWN-REGULATION

Modern medicine treats the disease and the symptoms too. The aim of ancient modalities is *swastha* or perfect wellbeing, besides the cure of the disease. It could in a sense be an idealist state of perfect health for which there is no limit. Contrast this with treating a patient for a given disease and that by itself being deemed to be an end in itself. It does not concern much with robust fitness thereafter. Ayurveda and yoga anticipate health problems and prep the person to mitigate future problems. They delay start of disease by addressing issues at the molecular level. The patient feels wellness and genetic balance even when some health issue remains to be resolved. In due course the expressions of the DNA change, even if the genetic code itself may remain unchanged. A couple of examples from *Dynamic DNA* will clarify the yoga-ayurveda approach.

Yoga and Ayurveda treat both the genotype and the phenotype, or the entire person, rather than the disease and the symptoms.[79] Their target first is the phenotype or the expression of the gene. For example, blond hair is an expression of the gene and is the phenotype. The gene does not have the code for brunette hair. This is the genotype. In the process of addressing the phenotype there is the confidence that genotype gets the message and lets the code either activate itself or stay inactive just as per the distinct intimations coming in from the conscious mind. The conscious mind has ways to communicate with the genotype: breathing, yogic exercises that fit the person, meditation, and diet. There could be others too, such as *sankalpa*! This could be true, for example, for someone with a genotype that increases the risk of atrial fibrillation. But it may not get expressed if the person is taking all the right steps to prevent the materialization of the threat inherent in the code.

One of the several cases of gene-level treatments using the yoga-ayurveda modality, cited in *Dynamic DNA,* refers to the randomized clinical trial with 201 black men and women with coronary heart disease. These subjects were called upon to practice TM. Among those that practiced TM, the risk of inflammation and cardiovascular disease was significantly reduced in expression (phenotype). TM reduced the risk of mortality, myocardial infarction, and stroke. On the other hand among those that did not practice TM, there were higher levels of expression in the two tumor suppressor genes.

Another specific example of the capabilities of Y-A intervention refers to a study of 30 men with low-risk prostate cancer who declined surgery, hormone therapy and radiation.[80] This study has been mentioned earlier. They opted for breathing exercises, meditation, low-fat, whole food, plant-based diet together with moderate exercises. The results were lower BP, Lower LDL cholesterol, lower prostate-specific antigen (PSA), lower weight and improved psychological functioning.

The main finding of the study was that relative telomere length increased from baseline by a median of 0·06 telomere to single-copy gene ratio (T/S); for the control group (-0·03 T/S units, -0·05 to 0·03, difference p=0·03). As has been noted earlier, telomerase is an enzyme that adds guanine rich repetitive sequences to telomeres and thus increases its length. After five years, telomerase activity had declined from baseline by 0·25 (-2·25 to 2·23) units in the lifestyle intervention group, and by 1·08 (-3·25 to 1·86) units in the control group (p=0·64), and was not associated with adherence to lifestyle changes (relative risk 0·93, 95% CI 0·72-1·20, p=0·57). Activity of 500 genes changed. 48 genes were upregulated and 452 genes were down-regulated or turned off. The latter included genes that were disease-promoting playing a critical role in tumor formation.[81, 82]

Meditational, yoga and ayurvedic techniques also go by the name of Mind Body Interventions (MBIs) which are known to improve physical and mental health. Clinical studies involving MBIs are not too many. One study reported that MBIs do downregulate nuclear factor kappa B pathway.[83] Chronic stress has the opposite effect on gene expressions. What it implies is that there could be a reduced risk of diseases caused/aided by inflammation. This study included both clinical and non-clinical samples, without much significance attached to research design. The authors encouraged more research so that the molecular mechanism of how the gene expressions are up or down regulated can be clearly understood.

When it is clinically proved that genes can be coaxed to activate or deactivate themselves, or up or down regulate themselves through simple yoga and/or ayurveda techniques, there is much skepticism, if not ridicule. The Ornish et al study mentioned earlier,[84] with its baffling results put down such skepticism. In this study of thirty men with low-risk prostate cancer opted for yoga-ayurveda alternative instead of the conventional radiation, surgery and radiation. Instead they routinely engaged themselves in a) breathing exercises b) meditation c) low-fat, whole-food plant based diet and d) moderate exercise. The results were: lower-prostate-specific antigen, lower blood pressure, lower LDL (bad) cholesterol, better psychological functioning, and also lower weight to boot. There was a change in activity of 500 genes as stated above, 48 genes up-regulated and 452 genes down-regulated. These 452 genes included disease promoting genes that played a critical role in tumor formation.

The Amazing Cellular World

Human body is made up of trillions of cells. Each cell is composed of cytoskeleton, cytoplasm, Golgi, lysosomes, organelles, mitochondria, nucleus, ribosomes and many more. Cells make up the structure of the human body and there are many different types of them: immune cells, neurons, muscle cells, cartilage cells, skeletal cells, pancreatic cells, white blood cells, red blood cells, platelets and so forth. Each one of those types is named according to their varied functions. Cells convert food into nutrients and convert nutrients into energy.

Hereditary materials are embedded into the nano-dimensions of the nucleus of the cells. True to its name, the nucleus is the command center in a cell, and issues directions to the cell to breed, nurture, mature, divide up and even undergo apoptosis, atrophy and mortality. Most importantly, the nucleus houses the DNA or the deoxyribonucleic acid which is the delivery service for the determinants of a person's future, the biological information or the hereditary material that is implanted in it.

Human and organic cells need instructions, inherent guidelines or codes to function the way they are supposed to and produce the materials like proteins from bio-sugars in the cells. These guidelines are contained in the DNA. Inherited characteristics are found in the DNA. For convenience we just think of them as instructions for making proteins from sugars. When you peep inside the nucleus we see chromatin and inside the chromatin we have the DNA and we can see its structure too. The DNA has smaller units called monomers or nucleotides which replicate themselves in a sequence. The three parts of a nucleotide are the phosphate group, a sugar (or deoxyribose) and a nitrogen (N) base, which has actually four (N) bases: ACTG or adenine, cytosine, thymine and guanine. TA and CG partner themselves always that way, as stated in the complementary base pairing rule.[85] They are the rungs of the double helix ladder attached to the phosphate bases at the two ends. AG are purines and CT are pyrimidines which are slanted to form a spiral helix. They were codiscovered in double spiral helix shape by Watson, Crick, Wilkins and Franklin who pieced the structure together.

Both the nucleus and mitochondria have DNA. DNA however is wrapped up in chromosomes in the nucleus. Mitochondrial DNA (mtDNA) has the genetic materials implanted in 37 genes. In the proper functioning of mitochondria each one of these genes plays a critical part. For instance, 13 of the genes issue instructions for making enzymes which are essential for oxidative phosphorylation which is the process for producing ATP or adenosine triphosphate using simple sugars. ATP is the source of energy for the cells. The other 24 genes issue the instructions needed for molecules like transfer RNA (tRNA) and ribosomal RNA (rRNA) which help convert protein building blocks into functioning proteins. The only way a person gets the mtDNA are from the mother through the egg cell.

ATGC Arrangement

In what order ATGC are arranged regulate the genetic code or the DNA instructions. The number of ATGC permutations can be four raised to the power of four (4^4) = 256. However human DNA instruction book or what is known as the genome for every human contains something like 3 billion bases or ATGC base pairs. The bases reside in 23 pairs of chromosomes. These very long chromosomes cannot be fitted into the nucleus without some unique coiling. The nucleus of the cells is somewhat crammed.[86] Nucleotides, to repeat, are organic molecules with a sugar molecule (nucleoside) on one side and a phosphate on the other, while the base serves as a rung in the ladder. A and T (in bases ATGC) pair together as a base as do G and C.

There is a sizzling discussion in advanced countries about the role of genetic modification as a solution to congenital or inherited problems in human health. The chapter on Yoga and Cancer brings up the question of genetic mutation or typos in genetic code that can be addressed by genetic engineering, or may be finagling. In some sectors the discussion is both brash and in other quarters it is cautious and mindful of the hazards of such genetic procedures that could be analogous to opening up several Pandora boxes at the same time. Green activists are vehement in their opposition to meddling with gene codes even in food items like carrots, peas, primroses, rice, onions, tomatoes, and others, including in the animal world like rats, mice, pigs, sheep, cats, dogs, primates and even fruit flies, leave alone in humans. This antagonism is well known. The most vocal and rational arguments against GMOs are those of Vandana Shiva. She is against industrial farming with heavy reliance on limited resources of the planet including water, and heavy use of pesticides, chemical fertilizers, and fossil fuels. She is all for organic ways of farming like in the good old days and for use of original seeds, not GMO seeds which leads to intellectual-property rights for seeds and 'seed dictatorship.' She thinks that even with the best of intentions one can still harm humanity and the planet.[87] The increasing food needs of the planet can be met through conventional seeds and farming methods.

In many countries it is also criminal to try alter human genes or "play God." In November 2018 a Chinese researcher He Jiankui and his two partners recruited couples and intentionally infected the fathers with HIV virus. He then modified a key gene in human embryos with the help of CRISPR technology to confer resistance to HIV. He and his two partners believed that descendants of children born with the modified genes may not have HIV. After his announcement of his genetic modification in real life, he was sentenced for three-years in prison together with a 3 million Chinese Yuan ($429,000) fine.[88] Nevertheless, scientists have been asking that genetic modifications should be one of the options on the table for almost incurable genetic diseases such as sickle-cell anemia or cystic fibrosis. A precondition for issue of permission for such research is the adherence to strict safety criteria.[89] Protest has not prevented advances in gene alterations. Microorganisms are very much in play. Gene reports about one's own gene make up are available from companies like Genes are Us and 23andme. Eugenics has led to biotech and from there you have biochemicals and biologicals, one of which is insulin. There are corporate businesses built on genetics like Biotech and Biogen.

While there are diseases that need to be addressed genetically, a vast majority of other medical issues are not inherited and so all modalities known to man and known to be adept in resolving contentious health issues need to be pressed into service. In the following part these possibilities are explored.

Yoga and Epigenetics

Much of this yoga research work is for the purpose of dealing with situations that naturally arise on account of certain life styles, diets, cultural, economic, political and religious practices or folklores and their like. For instance, one of the health issues that falls into this category is the DNA based categorization of people of Indian origin as more prone to heart diseases. Then there is the case of prion (proteinaceous infectious disease)[90], a neurodegenerative disease said to be caused by misfolded proteins in the brain. This can be fatal, and there may be sudden death without apparently any reason. Till a magic remedy is found for prion disease, the best that people with misfolded proteins can do is practice yoga exercises, avoid hectic life styles, consume vegetarian foods, and avoid liquor and fried foods, and stay within safe weight ranges. Such a regime could reduce the risk of sudden events by not stimulating the mal-mutations in genes to act up. Be that as it may, without solid determination or sankalpa, life style changes and diet regimes are the hardest modify. Some folks cling on to the life style they used to, come what may. For this reason, the Ayurveda-Yoga regime could be the best defense against prion disease. Ayurveda and yoga, however, do not open any Pandora 's Box or a can of worms. To the contrary, yoga and ayurveda deploy ancient wisdom in dealing with genes. Yoga and ayurveda are becoming known as epigenetics radiating new age thinking about resolving health issues by making sure that the hereditary DNA material in us function as well as they should. Typos in the genetic code increase risks of mutations in human cancer suppressor genes such as breast cancer Type 1 (BRCA$_1$) and breast cancer Type 2 (BRCA$_2$). And so instead of protecting the host body from getting cancer, they will increase the risk of cancer. These two genes are created naturally to repair such typos by tackling the gene expressions and not by meddling with the genetic codes.

Yoga Prompts Genetic Expression Change

The gentle and natural ways of yoga and ayurveda involving changes in diet, lifestyle and meditation can bring about changes in gene expressions, turning them off or on. They can be down- or up-regulated to reduce the risk of adverse human events like cancer. Therefore Yoga and Ayurveda are more promising in mitigating human suffering. Much of the ill-health events in one's life are predetermined or preordained by the genetic code. But as oncologist Mukherjee[91] notes: Biology is not destiny. There is much that is prompted by the environmental factors. This is where phenotype plays a crucial role in altering the expressions. However they are not of much help in bringing up alterations in genotype. That too may one day come within the realm of possibility, but it is still a pipe dream at this juncture.

Yogic life style increases the chances of change in gene expression and reduction in the damage potential of mutations in their tracks. For long the informed view has been that 'cancer was some kind of an exogenous event – a virus or something that could be got rid of, but cancer genes are sitting inside of each and every one of our chromosomes waiting to be corrupted or activated." [92] If the life style, diet, and environment are not of the desired type, cancer gene or the mal-gene may come under environmental pressure to come off the sleeper cell and act up as per their very code. Such gene-triggered sickness or more serious event like cancer would then have to show up. If on the other hand the ecosystem for an individual is health-oriented, and devoid of stress and bumpy-jumpy life, unhealthy life styles, and on the other hand, is yoga and ayurveda-influenced, the mal- or mutated gene has less chance to act up and wreak havoc. It has more rationale to remain passive.

There are two types of gene therapy. In one case a section of DNA is implanted into any cell in the body. In the other almost similar therapy, a section of DNA is implanted into cells that are actually getting active on their own, to enrich them or make good any deficiency.

The jury is still out as regards safety or otherwise of gene implants. There are health risks in view of inflammation, toxicity and even cancer. It is not yet accepted as a viable option considering that evaluations are still in progress. Clinical trials have been confined to mice and animals like in the case of diabetes type 2 although success has been reported in reversing obesity and insulin resistance in mice.

Invoking Parasympathetics

One of the unique features of yoga, as has been repeated earlier, is its proficiency in invoking of the parasympathetic nervous system to handle routine illness of any kind, instead letting the sympathetic system to respond to a health crisis. On account of this exceptional feature, yogic techniques such as deep breathing and Shavasana are considered the best prophylactic for stress management as well as its alleviation. Stress is a major killer and if one can gain proficiency in reining it in through yogic practices, yoga's rationale would sparkle bright. Professionals in the area of genetics can make good use of yoga-ayurveda capabilities to enhance medical efforts to ameliorate health conditions and otherwise revamp wellness.

A second exceptional fact is yoga, as its very name connotes (*yuj* in Sanskrit means joining or yoking together) is creating an ambience for the mind and body to work in harmony. Mind disciplines the body and that creates a virtuous cycle of more harmony and more synergy. Yoga helps self-improvement on a continuous basis. Society would welcome such a wholesome person as an asset, an advantage and strength in sync with its own best interests to improve phenotype and better tackle genotype issues.

Chapter 10

Yoga and Heart

The Wonder that is Heart

Heart related diseases are the *Numero Uno* leading cause of death in America as well as in India and most other countries. One in four deaths is caused by it. 647,000 persons die each year from it. [93] But what do we make of Health and Human Services report about the 83,000 drug overdose deaths in the 12 months period ended June 2020, mainly driven by serious mental ill-health worsened by social distancing like Surgeon General Vivek Murthy says in his recent book Together? This was discussed in Chapter 6. The point is stress-based mental illness and COVID-19 are vying with heart and cancer ailments, inter alia, also of stress-origin. Cardiac issues are making a big dent on American resources. Appropriately enough, we discuss yoga intervention (YI) in cardiac diseases to check if such intervention makes sense in terms of amelioration of any heart disease or condition.

Cardiac Problems and the Yoga Remedy

The mind-boggling pump that the heart is can be fully comprehended only by learning all about it. The atriums, ventricles, the aorta, pulmonary vena cava, the sophisticated manner the one-way tricuspid and bicuspid aortal and other valves function, how the heart pumps CO_2-laden vein blood to the lungs and gets back oxygenated blood and circulates it to all parts of the body, the inbuilt pace maker on the right side of the heart with an AV node in the cardiac septum muscle and much more, are fascinating and all interested in health and wellness would do well to know about them. The ventricle valve shutting with a Lub sound and the aortic valve shutting with a Dub sound, (hence Lub-Dub) are worth listening to. Whether they were designed as such *ab initio* or just evolved into such startling intricacy makes no difference to the intense wonder the heart evokes as a critical human biomechanical component of the human body.

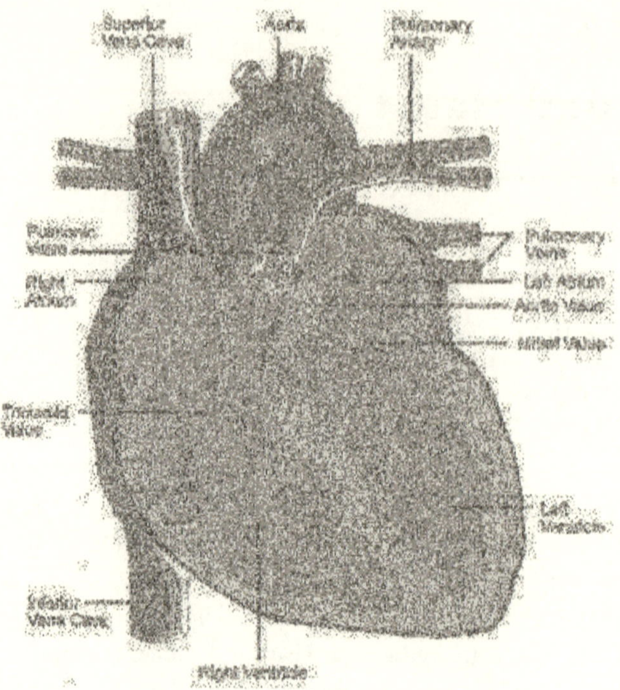

Fig 11: The Heart: A Cross-Sectional View
Source: nhlbi.nih.gov

Millions of people all over the world suffer from various kinds of heart problems, from minor conditions such as abnormal rhythms (arrhythmia) and angina all the way to the more serious problems such as heart attack, heart failure, hypertension, stroke and valve diseases. Cardiac disease, as noted above, is the number one cause of death at present. The promotion of activity that is wholesome for heart care cannot be stressed enough. Yoga has many remedial techniques to ameliorate heart conditions: abdominal and other breathing, meditation, shavasana (corpse pose), numerous stretching exercises, subtle mudras like the Shanmukhi, as well as krias, and bandhas. They prevent cardiac adverse events too.

But human nature being what it is, often takes the "if it ain't broke, don't fix it" approach to heart health. Until one has an attack, which is the term used for blockage of blood flow to the heart muscle, most people do not take any preemptive steps to guard against a weakening of the heart, let alone take steps to promote a strong sturdy heart. They believe that such a thing cannot happen to them even if they flout all the sound rules of wellness, such as emotionally getting stressed, being excessively anxious about something that affect their life style, overeating, or putting on weight and straining the heart. Some wait until cholesterol completely blocks the arteries, tissues lose oxygen and the heart muscle goes virtually dead.

Everybody knows that 'an ounce of prevention is better than a pound of cure' but not many care to practice it. As stated earlier, both in India and in America more and more people are becoming overweight (body-mass-index or BMI going above 25) or even obese with BMI exceeding 30. Overweight and obese persons, whose numbers are going up increase the risk for many diseases and health conditions. (Please see page 63 for data on overweight and obesity.)

Stress Cannot be Busted for Good!

Stress is the worst culprit for heart problems. There are two kinds of stress: a beneficial kind such as when we are eager and excited to meet our loved ones; and second, deleterious kind such as when you suddenly discover that you have just 30 minutes to complete an assignment when it requires at least three hours! That tense feeling you have when you are already late to catch a flight and there is a horrendous traffic jam on the road to the airport! Or like when we found out on September 2008 that a leading financial institution such as Lehman Brothers had filed for bankruptcy protection; or Merrill Lynch had sold itself to Bank of America; and we started wondering whether our lifetime nest egg earnings in our 401(k) accounts were safe! Nobody can be free from stress because of the very nature of the world in which we live. Through judicious choice, however, we can reduce our exposure to deleterious stress. But you can put out of your mind thoughts about eliminating stressful experiences all together unless you take to *sanyasa* or hermitage or total detachment *(or vairagya)* from the material world.

It is wise to learn about the health of one's own heart, such as optimal blood pressure and high blood pressure. Normal blood pressure is 120/80 for systolic and diastolic pressures, with accommodations for age. Blood pressure measurement is needed to determine if there is hypertension often caused by smoking, overweight, sedentary habits and lack of exercise, pregnancy in women, but most significantly, by a stressful life. On the other hand, low blood pressure, particularly in athletes could be indicative of good heart health, though it could hide other problems.

Early Studies Reveal Benefits of YI

Lifestyle modification incorporating yoga practices has benefitted patients to retard coronary artery disease (CAD). In a 2000 prospective, randomized controlled trial 42 men with angiographically proven CAD were randomized to control (n =21) and to YI group (n=21).[94] They were observed for a year. The Yoga group practiced yoga, controlled risk factors, including diet control and did moderate aerobic exercise. The control group was managed by conventional risk factor control and American Heart Association step I diet. The Yoga group registered significant reduction in the number of anginal episodes per week, improved exercise capacity and decreases in body weight. There were significant reductions in serum total cholesterol, LDL cholesterol, and triglyceride levels compared to the control group. There was less frequent use of revascularization procedures in the yoga group – such as one versus 8 patients, relative risk = 5.45; P = 0.01. There were significantly more lesions regressed (20% versus 2%) and less lesions progressed such as 5% as against 37% in the yoga group (chi-square = 24.9; P < 0.0001). The conclusion was yoga lifestyle intervention retards progression and increases regression of coronary atherosclerosis in patients with CAD.

A 2018 study studied efficacy of yoga-based lifestyle program (YLSP) in improving quality of life (QoL) and stress levels in patients 5 years after coronary artery bypass graft (CABG).[95] 300 patients posted for CABG in a Bengaluru hospital were randomized into YLSP and conventional life style program (CLSP) and were followed up for five years. Yoga therapy consisting of yama, niyama, asana, pranayama and meditation was brought to bear on YLSP and CLSP followed conventional rehabilitation. At the end of five years there were significant improvements in the YLSP as compared to the CLSP in mental health (P = 0.05), perceived stress (P = 0.01) and negative affect (NA) (P = 0.05). The WHO-QOL BREF showed improvements in physical health (P = 0.046), environmental health (P= 0.04), perceived stress (P= 0.001) and NA (P = 0.02). Positive affect improved significantly in the CLSP, but not in the YLSP. There were no revealed significant differences in the other domains of WHO-QOL-BREF, PANAS, and HADS.

Meta-Analysis of YI in Clinical Trials

One of the robust evidences of the beneficial impact of yoga interventions such as asanas, breathing exercises, meditation and ethical norms for cardiac problems is the meta-analysis consisting of 17 studies completed by Marshall Hagins.[96] This study showed that interventions such as asanas, breathing and meditation had clinically significant BP reduction such as 8 mm HG for systolic and 6 mm HG diastolic.

By following designated yoga practices, it is possible to train cardio-vascular (heart-lung) system to withstand greater amount of stresses and pressures of everyday life. For example simple stretching exercises such as hand, leg, and back stretches reduce anxiety levels and muscle tension. Breathing becomes more abdominal and regular. These bodily changes contribute to reduction of high blood pressure. Regular yoga practice reduces the risk of heart attack and also the chances of artery blockage.

In a 12-week long study the efficacy of Iyengar Yoga and Enhanced Usual Care (EUC) (somewhat like a control group) were compared to study their effect on 24-hour ambulatory BP in yoga-naïve adults with untreated prehypertension or Stage 1 hypertension. In the yoga group there were 26 participants and in the EUC group there were 31 participants. The results showed no difference in BP between the two groups at six and twelve weeks. 24-h systolic BP (SBP), diastolic BP (DBP) and mean arterial pressure (MAP) went down in the EUC group by 5, 3 and 3 mmHg respectively from the baseline at 6 weeks (P <. 05) but they were not significant at 12 weeks. In contrast the YI group 24 h SBP went down by 6 mmHg at 12 weeks compared to the baseline (P =. 05). Also 24 DBP (P<.01) and MAP (P<.05) decreased significantly by 5 mmHg. There were no differences in the catecholamine or cortisol metabolism as an explanation for the decrease in BP in the IY group. The study concluded that 12 weeks of IY resulted in clinically meaningful improvements in 24-h SBP and DBP.[97]

In one of the comprehensive studies Anupama Tyagi and Marc Cohen (2013) looked into yoga-HTP associations and results over four decades and reported that studies of yoga interventions together with numerous experimental designs have consistently reported reduction in BP as well as reductions in CVD risk factors such as lipid profile, glycemic index, weight and HR. Of 120 studies covered by Tyagi et al, 23 (including 12 RCTs) reported no change in BP.

Hypertension (HPT) is defined as Systolic Blood Pressure (SBP) persistently greater than 140 and Diastolic Blood Pressure greater than 90 and HPT is a world-wide problem affecting one billion persons. It accounts for 13% of deaths, and disability-adjusted-life-years (DALYs) and seven million premature deaths annually. If current trends continue without discontinuities, by 2025 one in three adults over 20 years of age will be suffering from HTP: or a staggering total of 1.56 billion will have this complaint.[98]

Research performed over the past 40 years with various yoga interventions, including studies with different experimental designs, consistently reported reductions in BP together with reductions in other CVD risk factors such as lipid profile, glycemic index, weight, and HR. The BP reductions reported with yoga were found in diverse populations, including both hypertensive and normotensive populations. It would be commonplace among the unfit as well athletic individuals, in adolescents as well as the elderly. Yoga was also found to reduce BP in participants taking antihypertensive medications. Yoga helped reduce medication use while maintaining reduced BP.

Yoga Guidelines to Reduce BP

One of the highlights of the Tyagi et al Review was that on account of heterogeneity of yoga exercises and practices (which would serve as confounding variables used in the interventions) it was not possible to list accurately the yoga exercises that helped reduce BP, though shavasana, breathing, meditation are mentioned in most of the studies. This heterogeneity study suggested clinical trials using specific yogic exercises to make accurate guidelines regarding practices that would definitely reduce BP.

A 2016 study brought out significant differences in BP of females in the age group of 26 - 40 years between pre- and post-yoga intervention and between this experimental group and the control group. The experimental group followed yoga protocols for six months. For the control group general warm up exercises were prescribed and games were played for the same period. In the case of the experimental group there was significant change in DBP from pre-test 72.36 to post-test 93.72. The corresponding DBP data for the control group was pre-test 74.28 and post-test 72.24. The study concluded that there were significant changes in BP for the experimental group for both SBP and DBP[99]

One half of 4000 heart attack survivors in India participated in a yoga rehabilitation program and the other half in conventional cardiac rehabilitation program which is uncommon in India. The experimental group did gentle yoga asanas and protocols and the other half received standard care. The conclusion was that yoga based rehabilitation was a safe alternative to conventional rehabilitation.[100]

Yoga, Meditation and CVD

Till about the fifties or even later, the word Yoga connoted not just the asana exercises, breathing, mudras and other kriyas, but also the post pranayama stages of pratyahara or withdrawal from topics or subjects not relevant to one's lifetime goals, dharana or focus on topics of relevance to one's life, dhyana or meditation on the topic of interest at any one given time, and samadhi which was the ultimate goal of becoming a philosopher of life without attachment of any kind or being connected to anything or any idea like we saw under Kundalini Chakra. This was the complete view of yoga, as a way of life. Meditation was an integral part of yoga. Of late meditation has acquired a separate status which could pigeon-hole it and deny the benefits of holistic or integrated yoga to meditators.

Yogic meditation or the ability to scan our thoughts, their antecedents, their reverberations and picking up the most optimum choice of direction for those thoughts or the course of action, is perhaps more rational than most people think it is. Meditation is a cool reflection on what has happened, where any particular matter stands and ideally or desirably should be the direction in which it should move further. This is a kind of checklist of correct sequence of steps for any activity. The final outcome should be one of peace with oneself, one's life, one's ecosystem, one's outlook or philosophy of life, a constant reconciliation with matters as they stand, or bold steps needed to put things right if well within one's faculty and resources. Such pre-meditated steps are anytime better than unpreparedness or, being another manifestation of Don Quixote's expedition against the wind mills. Not surprisingly, the science and rationality underlying meditation has been recognized the world over.

The American Heart Association has issued a Scientific Statement on Meditation and Cardiovascular Risk Reduction. In their study that forms the foundation for the official policy statement, the focus is only on sitting meditation and not on other related techniques and life styles associated with yoga, viz., mudras, asanas, Yamas or the rules of conduct in dealing with the external ecosystem such as non-violence, truth and non-covetousness, Niyamas or norms for self-conduct and attitude with oneself such as cheerfulness, mental and physical cleanliness, life-long learning and so forth. The reason given for the focus on meditation alone is that bringing in all other factors would result in confounding. One would be at a loss to identify and isolate the benefits of meditation alone and recommend it for adoption as a complementary and inexpensive modus operandi for CVD risk reduction. It is therefore essential to define meditation and what yoga baggage it brings with it in order to be able to estimate its outcomes.

AHA states that neurophysiological and neuroanatomical studies have demonstrated that meditation could have long-standing effects on the brain, with attendant collateral consequences for the physiological basal state including reduction in CVD risk. Also mentioned are physiological response to stress, smoking cessation, BP reduction, insulin resistance and metabolic syndrome, ischemia, endothelial function and others.[101] Meditation is a "….novel and inexpensive intervention that can contribute to the primary and secondary prevention of cardiovascular disease…" The benefits of meditation have been documented widely. AHA also criticizes that the quality of the studies and the quantity of evidence from those studies remain modest. Despite that limitation, AHA concedes the benefits of meditation on CVD risk reduction and recommends its use as an "…… adjunct to guideline-directed" CVD reduction. It hints that there could be lifestyle modification. This does take into account the fact of American individualism and its ideation that do not easily appreciate the rationale of stooping to conquer. This prominent American characteristic gets in the way of embracing meditation and is unlikely to be entertained by conformity suggested by an endorsement by an authority like the AHA.

YI: More Clinical Evidence

A meta-analysis on the role of yoga on modifying risk factors for cardiac diseases published in 2014 took into account 37 randomized control trials in a systematic review and 32 of the same in a meta-analysis.[102] The results buoyed up yoga community. The study concluded that there was significant reduction in body mass index ($-0.77\,kg/m^2$ (95% confidence interval -1.09 to -0.44)), systolic blood pressure ($-5.21\,mmHg$ (-8.01 to -2.42)), low-density lipoprotein cholesterol ($-12.14\,mg/dl$ (-21.80 to -2.48)), and high-density lipoprotein cholesterol ($3.20\,mg/dl$ (1.86 to 4.54)). Significant changes were seen in body weight ($-2.32\,kg$ (-4.33 to -0.37)), diastolic blood pressure ($-4.98\,mmHg$ (-7.17 to -2.80)), total cholesterol ($-18.48\,mg/dl$ (-29.16 to -7.80)), triglycerides ($-25.89\,mg/dl$ (-36.19 to -15.60)), and heart rate (-5.27 beats/min (-9.55 to -1.00)), but not fasting blood glucose ($-5.91\,mg/dl$ (-16.32 to 4.50)) nor glycosylated hemoglobin (-0.06% Hb (-0.24 to 0.11)). Yoga was also found to have an impact on smoking abstinence according to one of these studies. This is promising evidence of yoga improving cardiometabolic health.

More Meta-Analysis Evidence

Yet another interesting meta-analysis of yoga intervention in cardiac diseases is a 2014 German study unequivocally stating that regular practice of yoga could have clinically important effect on risk factors for CVD.[103]

What comes in for endorsement is that yoga is a combination of exercises, breathing and relaxation techniques contributing to the reduction of biological risk factors. Cramer H et al included 44 controlled trials with a total of 3168 subjects. Some subjects were healthy, but in the case of others it included patients with comorbidities such as diabetes, hypertension, prehypertension, metabolic syndrome, obesity, dyslipidemia, and impaired insulin resistance. The improvements that the yoga intervention group registered over the control group were the following:

- Systolic BP: mean difference, –5.85 mm Hg (95% CI, –8.81 to –2.89).
- Diastolic BP: –4.12 mm Hg (95% CI, –6.55 to –1.69).
- Heart rate: –6.59 bpm (95% CI, –12.89 to –0.28).
- Respiratory rate: –0.93 breaths/minute (95% CI, –1.7 to –0.15).
- Waist circumference: –1.95 cm (95% CI, –3.01 to –0.89).
- Waist/hip ratio: –0.02 (95% CI, –0.03 to 0).
- Total cholesterol: –13.09 mg/dL (95% CI, –19.6 to –6.59).
- HDL: 2.94 mg/dL (95% CI, 0.57-5.31).
- Very low-density lipoprotein: –5.7 mg/dL (95% CI, –7.36 to –4.03).
- Triglycerides: –20.97 mg/dL (95% CI, –28.61 to –13.32).
- HbA1c: –0.45% (95% CI, –0.87 to –0.02).
- Insulin resistance: –0.19 (95% CI, –0.3 to –0.08).

In addition, compared with exercise, yoga was associated with improved HDL (mean difference, 3.7 mg/dL; 95% CI, 1.14-6.26).

Not all trials reported safety-related information, but those that did, did not find serious adverse events for yoga participants.

German researchers found many lacunae in the research protocols of studies included in the Meta analysis. Some of them were: selection bias because random sequence generation was not adhered to for picking the studies. There was no masking of outcome assessment in the case of some 31 studies. None of the effects in the mea-analysis could be regarded as a robust outcome. Nevertheless, yoga being safe with little side-effects, YI was perhaps endorsed for improving CVD risks.

Lifestyles Unmodifiable?

Most people like in India or America are highly individualistic and refuse to accept any suggestions for modification of lifestyles even if it is shown that the lifestyle they are adhering to is harmful for a healthy heart or a healthy life. Smoking or drinking beer for example, are known to be bad for the lungs and for keeping weights down. They have grown into well-practiced habits in almost all advanced countries which are mimicked in developing countries as signs of progressiveness. Knowing something to be bad for health and still sticking to a unhealthy habit or lifestyle causes psychological stress because of contradictory oxymoronic behavior.

Lifestyles are nonmodifiable for some folks, come what may: obesity, high blood sugar, hypertension, unhappiness or whatever. The undeclared thought is that there are always magic bullet treatments and medications to take care of any health problem, however much acute, complex or expensive. The behavioral matters relate to food, leisure, entertainment, workloads, commuting to work, following specific guidelines for any one of the above. There is nonchalance and denials all the way even when egregious evidence to the contrary is strewn all over, or right in the face. Most recommendations to manage hypertension are confined to diet and exercise and not much to lifestyle changes.[104]

Thus while there is ample evidence to prove effectiveness of yoga practices for reducing hypertension, guidelines for treating hypertension do not refer to yoga thanks to a) unfamiliarity with yoga practice and b) the heterogeneity of yoga practices and differing claims. Fortunately, however, the quality of clinical trials of late seem to be meeting standard criteria such as those of the FDA or the Cochrane Reviews.

Variability in Effect and Effectiveness Ascribed to Asanas

New research has highlighted the need to view both the effect and efficacy of yoga exercises more mindfully instead of regarding them all as having almost the same outcomes and having the same effectiveness. A 2014 carefully designed study has confirmed that all asanas and yoga practices are not the same whether in terms of needed impact on physical/psychological conditions and in terms of the efficacy of the same. Also the timing of the exercise is of consequence. For instance, the study showed that shavasana by itself, would not be as effective as when it is followed by performance of asanas.[105]

The study proceeded to record heart rate (HR), systolic pressure (SP), and diastolic pressure (DP), blood pressure (BP), with the help of noninvasive blood pressure (NIBP) apparatus in 22 healthy young subjects, before and after the performance of Dhanurasana (DA), Vakrasana (VA) (both sides), Janusirasasana (JSA) (both sides), Matsyasana and Shavasana for 30 seconds. The researchers noted the HR and BP scores during supine recovery at intervals of 2, 4, 6, 8, and 10 minutes. Repeated Measure ANOVA was used for statistical analysis. The heart rate and BP were found to be significantly different for the different asanas and for the interval recuperation period. The details given in the study were that the decrease of SP after VA (right side) (VA-R) was significantly greater than Shavasana (4th, 6th, and 8th min) and JSA (left side) (JSA-L) at 6th and 8th min. DP decreased significantly after performing JSA-L compared to VA-R at the 6th and 8th min. Dhanurasana increased the heart rate significantly more than other asanas. This is attributed to the difficulty in performing and the response of the sympathetic nervous system to the effort. The study found that the effect of shavasana is more obvious after doing the asanas, as compared to relaxation in shavasana *per se*. Pre-shavasana exercise activity brings about a normalization and homeostatic effect of the autonomous nervous system and thus there is healthier de-activation during such shavasana.

The foregoing notes about effectiveness and actual outcomes of each asana or yoga exercise being different are of particular significance when prescribing yoga regimen and the sequence of yoga asanas or mudras or breathing exercises and others in the yoga package to patients.

*Clinical evidence is being offered in the following chapter on effectiveness of **Yoga Intervention (YI) for Cancer**. Besides such clinical evidence, there are several references to anecdotal evidence, besides views of researchers.*

Chapter 11

Yoga and Cancer

What is Cancer?

Uncontrolled proliferation of generally abnormal cells in a living body manifests itself as cancer. Normal cells have defined physiological, anatomical and other biochemical functions to perform and are needed for the sustenance of life and body. On the other hand, cancer cells are relatively larger, needless, purposeless and abnormal with varied shapes of nuclei. They divide themselves up in an anarchic way and their sizes and shape are disorderly. They have no normal features. They happen, inter alia, due to stress, trauma and mutations in genes. The abnormal cells, unlike the benign variety, tend to spread to other parts of the human body. Whenever one speaks of cancer there is also a chat about tumors, benign or malignant. The former stays put in a part of the body, but the latter spreads.

No one wants these abnormal cells in any living body. They are not the outcome of typical and regular embedded instructions in a person's DNA or something initiated by way of planned intervention of any kind. Different parts of the body can have cancerous growth, like skin cancer, or carcinoma. There are different names for cancers of parts of the body like breast, lung, lymphatic cell, renal cell, prostate, colorectal, thyroid, uterine, and so forth. When blood cells have cancer, it is leukemia.

Cells without a Purpose

Normal cells have a purpose or they are created for a reason like neurons in the brain to generate electrical impulses that combine and become thoughts, or alveoli in lungs that promote the vital gas exchange, or parietal cells, podocytes and mesangial cells in the kidneys that separate toxic stuff that is drained out through urine, or the alpha cells in pancreas (islets of Langerhans) that generate insulin or glucagon. But the wretched cancer cells have no purpose and multiply like crazy!

In 2020 there will be about 1.8 million new cancer cases according to the American Cancer Society and the number of deaths about 606,520, which is approximately a third of the new cases. The number of cancer survivors is currently about six million in America. This number is also increasing.

There are different causes or risk factors that could provide the hospitable environs for cancer. If we know the causes of cancer, we can try prevention more scientifically. However, it is matter-of-fact to remember that anyone risk factor can be more of a root-cause for one person and less so, or no cause at all for another. Taking all related factors into account, it would appear that anxieties and stress are the most principal cause, the *agent provocateurs*. Those at peace with themselves are at much lower risk of being victims of this awful predicament, second largest cause of death.

The biochemistry and nervous system of an apprehensive or restless person are significantly different from when such a person is calm and cheerful. There is much tension and the heart rate goes up, the systolic and diastolic pressures would be way above the normal 120-70. That is true of the heart rate too, way above the normal 72 per minute. Emotions and feelings seem out of whack. Other symptoms could be body aches, headaches, constipation or diarrhea, tendency to constantly eat, smoke, drink, and indulge in unhealthy activity. It is somewhat encouraging that there is growing awareness today, if not consensus, that for disturbed and troubled cancer-affected persons, yoga offers the inexpensive but effective medicine and therapy. The clinical evidence for this assessment is offered here.

Smoking: A Cordial Invite for Cancer

Tobacco smoke was classified late in 1992 as one of the most dangerous cancer-causing 'Group A' carcinogen.[106] Tobacco smoke is known to consist of over 4000 chemical compounds and 60 known carcinogens, half of the compounds occurring naturally in green tobacco and the other half when tobacco is burnt. Tobacco smoke includes carbon monoxide, hydrogen cyanide, benzene, formaldehyde, nicotine, phenol, polycyclic aromatic hydrocarbons (PAHs) and tobacco-specific nitrosamines (TSNAs).

Smoking of all kinds is another reason for cancer, in particular lung cancer, with the lungs exposed to smoke. It could be mainstream smoke, e-cigarettes, vapid pod smoking, or secondary or sidestream smoke which is equally or more hazardous. Wood-smoke from burning wood for cooking purposes or burning coal for cooking in choolahs are also carcinogenic. Next to tobacco smoke, genetic codes, rather the typos in them, are another risk factor for hereditary cancer. In epidemiological studies there is comparison of people that have some form of cancer with those that don't have any. The lifestyles are contrasted and broad conclusions are drawn as to why some suffer and others are not at all affected by this frightful predicament. Smoking and hereditary factors show up well in these. The National Cancer Institute lists the following as physiological risk factors for cancer: age, alcohol, cancer causing chemical substances, inflammation, diet, hormones, immunosuppression, infectious agents, radiation, sunlight and tobacco.[107] Persistent anxieties and stress are, as stated above psychosomatic *agent provocateurs* of cancer.

Unfortunately, humans are predisposed to commit oversight such as knowledgeably leading stressful lives, overeating, consuming wrong foods, overindulging in pleasures, intemperate drinking of alcohol beverages, smoking, living in polluted cities and environments, over-medicating oneself and their like. How deliberately such wrong activity is pursued has to be seen to be believed. It is like people wanting to live on Skid Row just for the heck, with no goals on *terra firma*, and that they didn't choose to be born of their own volition! Thus, there is an increase in vulnerability to not just cancers, but also to numerous other diseases. People are overwhelmed by anxiety and stress caused sometimes by the dizzying speed of societal change and transformation. In this state of mind, the range of movement of the limbs of the body unhappily decreases. Aging occurs faster. The downward spiral of the functionality of endocrine glands begins, with possible onset of numerous morbidities including diabetes. And healthy life span gets shorter and shorter.

There is always the wisdom of yoga encouraging us to make healthy choices for robust health. Regular daily yoga practices and lifestyles reduces the risk of falling sick for any reason. Even if sickness comes due to a variety of factors like pollution of food, water or air, the body's immune mechanism kicks in proficiently, homeostasis sets in and the body is restored to normal health rapidly. A yoga person may recover from a cold, cough or fever after 12 to 24 hours of rest; whereas other persons may take a few days to recover. Travel and vacation periods are particularly stressful in our times, and it is all the more crucial that time is set aside for yoga and relaxation to enable the body and mind to attune themselves to the new environment. How hard is it to have deep abdominal breathing as one's default breathing?

Yoga Helps Cancer Person Scuba-Dive

Besides many research studies in India, one of the earliest studies on YI in cancer was by Joseph CD (1983.)[108] This was not a randomised study with experimental and control groups, but a simple one, just more than a pilot study. The results were not in the form of pre and post-intervention assessments, but more in the form of self-reported assessment by the patients. The study highlighted that YI helped appetite improvement 22%, sleep 22%, and bowel habits 26%. YI helped generate a feeling of more peace and tranquility 20% in the post-yoga intervention period. The sample consisted of 50 outpatient or ambulatory cancer patients visiting the cancer center for radiation therapy. The YI sessions lasted 90 minutes and were in batches of 10-12 patients. The yoga instruction consisted mainly of relaxation exercises without vigorous and exhausting exercises.

A 2005 study by Bower JE et al [109] made a review of nine studies, including the one by Joseph CD mentioned above. All nine of them dealt with yoga intervention in cancer patients and survivors. What was perhaps having a confounding effect was the "all-purpose" nature of YI as well as the heterogeneity of YI. The studies also did not provide details of the nature of yoga sessions: asanas, breathing, mudras, doses of yoga exercises, their nature and others. Not surprisingly, the results were wide-ranging, covering different types of cancer, stages of disease, and at what stage in the treatment trajectory the patients were. The Bower study also recommended more targeted YI such as for dealing with fatigue in breast cancer patients with Sethubandasana. The study was however, unequivocal in concluding that yoga was both a feasible and efficient intervention for wide range of cancers including lymphoma, breast and prostate.

Yoga as Complementary Treatment

One of the well-known cancer specialists that believed in complementary, as opposed to alternative, healing systems was Dr. William Fair, mentioned earlier on page 24. That is to say, Fair, a specialist in prostate cancer, Sloan Memorial Kettering Institute, did not believe in substituting standard medicine for cancer with alternative medicine or treatment, but wanted to logically try complementary medicine when in 1995 he was diagnosed with colon cancer. The difference between alternative and complementary medicine is, in the former case, there is substitution of conventional medicine, whereas in complementary medicine a new treatment or medicine is used along with regular treatment. Fair submitted himself to conventional chemotherapy and surgery. It recurred in 1997. Again he endured more of the same. He also concluded that there was little chance of a cure, somewhat of a contra-sankalpa, losing resoluteness in the context of being pragmatic. "My choices were limited — another risky operation, extensive radiation and experimental chemotherapy." A complementary medicine center was opened and in its brochure Dr. Fair wrote "Knowing these treatments could be very toxic and debilitating, I set out on my own to investigate approaches outside conventional medicine that I felt would preserve my quality of life and perhaps slow the progression of the disease."

Fair began with rigorous yoga, exercise, prayer and meditation as well as making changes in his diet and taking herbal treatments – protocols he had earlier rejected as "touchy-feely nonsense." Nevertheless, he felt better. The tumors shrank thanks to the unconventional therapies. But cancer recurred and yet many were surprised he lived that long after coming down with colon cancer.[110] Yoga may not have cured him of cancer, but it allowed him to continue living fully, improved quality of life, and helped manage his cancer with less pain. Fair wrote in the *New Yorker* magazine that vigorous practice of yoga helped him to gain more energy. He was able to see more patients, write research papers for professional journals such as *Alternative Therapies in Health and Medicine,* and *Molecular Urology,* spend more time with his family and even go scuba-diving!

Today there is unmistakable progress towards holistic and interdisciplinary therapies that combine best practices in different health care modalities, which for convenience has been christened complementary and alternative medicine or CAM. As an example, take women with breast cancer: in 80% such cases CAM therapies such as yoga are used to overcome side effects of treatment.[111] In a 2012 meta-analysis study by Buffart LM et al[112] significant findings were noted in regard to YI in the case of breast cancer patients. The study found large reductions in distress, anxiety and depression (d = –0.69 to –0.75), moderate reductions in fatigue (d = –0.51), moderate increases in general quality of life, emotional function and social function (d = 0.33 to 0.49), and a small increase in functional well-being (d = 0.31). Effects on physical function and sleep were small and not significant.

Breast cancer and lymphoma patients underwent a supervised yoga program which included asanas, breathing techniques and shavasana relaxation and meditation or "dhyana." There was thus preliminary support for YI in cancer situations. The meta-analysis of randomized clinical trials (RCTs) showed that there was "strong beneficial effects" on distress, anxiety and depression. The conclusion from the same evidence was that there was "moderate effect on fatigue, general Health Related QoL, emotional function and social function, small effects on functional wellbeing and no significant effects on physical function and sleep disturbances."

To avoid publication bias offered below is a 2012 study on YI for fatigue mainly in cancer patients concluding that yoga did not have a perceptible effect. Fatigue or exhaustion is both mental and physical. Repetitively done jobs, especially routinely, without much enthusiasm, could sap one's energy, both in a subjective and practical sense. One kind of exhaustion comes from medical routines – the tiresome protocols, taking medications, undergoing chemotherapy, radiation, the side effects, performing exercises, eating the same diet and facing the same tedious or dreary environment. There are exercises that are energizing and they help a person get over exhaustion and keep functioning till the purpose of any action is accomplished. One study by way of a meta-analysis of 19 clinical studies (total n = 948) discussed a variety of yoga exercises for persons suffering from cancer, multiple sclerosis, dialysis, chronic pancreatitis, fibromyalgia, asthma and others who were healthy.[113] The study found that yoga had only a small positive effect on fatigue (SMS = 0.27, 59% CI = 0.23-0.31.) The conclusion was that the effects of yoga interventions on fatigue were only slight, particularly in the case of cancer patients. While there is a general feel that yoga has therapeutic effects, this meta-analysis could not show the powerful effect of yoga on patients' fatigue and anyone can see why: there is considerable heterogeneity with several morbidities put together with cancer.

On Yoga-Ayurveda (YA) therapy

Over the past 20 years there have been far-reaching enhancements in the effectiveness in alternative and complementary medicine for cancer. These advances were highlighted at the International Conference on Integrative Medicine – Role of Yoga and Ayurveda in the Management of Cancer and Palliative Care held at Harvard Medical School's Joseph Martin Conference Center, June 22-24, 2018. Details of the discussions and deliberations at this Conference are available online.[114] Among other things, it looked into the costs of cancer drugs, outcomes of clinical yoga interventions for cancer, dietary planning, herbascuticals, meditation, deep abdominal breathing and pranayama, Ayurvedic interventions and related matters. Comparative performance-effectiveness and cost-effectiveness too were considered. The aim, *inter alia*, of the meet was one of highlighting the capabilities of Ayurveda and Yoga techniques and thereby help them gain more currency as efficient, if not sounder means to deploy against cancer and other grave threats to wellness. What follows are some of the keynotes of the YA Conference without details of speakers and their specific research results which are available in the source mentioned in endnote #114 above.

Keynotes of 2018 Conference

Chemotherapy is expensive and painful and often ineffective, with a probability of relapse. Prevention is any time preferable by strengthening the immune system through unremitting practice of yoga. Also, yoga helps manage cancer effects better. There is good reason to pay more attention to what yoga can do before cancer, and also for cancer survivors. This is particularly more urgent for patients that are not likely to benefit much from chemotherapy.

Cancer drugs are expensive. They can shrink even well off patients into "financial orphans," thanks to corporate concerns for return on Investments (ROI) whereas herbal options are amazingly affordable. Second, herbal options have proved more effective in terms of remission in severity of cancer. Invariably it boosts the patient's immune makeup, the first defense against cancer cells. The early battles against cancer are won right there. There are advantages to an integrated therapeutic program for dealing with any chronic sickness. Rationally speaking, in the Yoga-Ayurveda (YA) system, less is more. There is virtue in austerity and under-treatment rather than the other way around. Austerity perks up homeostatic and lymphatic rigors in the whole system which transmutes into a more holistic system. Evidence is also coming up that genes can be subjected to down- or upregulation, as needed, through simple method of Yoga guided meditation by the patient. See Chapter Chapter 9: Yoga and Genes.

Merits of Yoga Life Style

Under the yoga approach to cancer management, it is not a case of battling cancer, but one of enabling a person to live with it, if one cannot get rid of it. In a way Ayurveda is comprehensible to the west for it talks of Ayuh or longevity. When there is fusion of the three dimensions of human personality of body, mind and spirit, the whole becomes greater than the sum of the parts due to synergy and organic interaction. The transcendental aspect begins to emerge. This condition is beyond the senses. Yoga meditation too can get there. Yoga and ayurvedic life style are transforming. In this milieu, yoga health and meditation can touch DNA. What need emphasis for cancer-affected persons are three specifics: a) Ayurvedic lifestyle, diet and nutrition, herbs, stress management and environmental factors help manage epigenetic factors b) YA is the science of epigenetics, affecting phenotype, and may be, on some future date, genotype too. It is a complete and comprehensive science of life. And c) It is possible to create a cancer-free body integrating YA with the health care system over a period of time.

There is evidence that good and sacrosanct sound (Sama Veda incantation) decreases malignant cell growth. It showed a 25.3% in reduction in brain malignant glioma cell growth, 16.9% reduction in breast adenocarcinoma, 19.9% reduction in colon adenocarcinoma, 22.4% in lung carcinoma, and so forth on listening to Sama Veda (p-value < 0.005, ANOVA). [115] (See Table 9 below.) Some of the work in epigenetics is made possible with the aid of electro-photo imaging (EPI) which reads photon emissions from the finger tips. Yoga too uses the same paradigm of neuroplasticity to reverse any abnormal condition.

Just as good quality of life, with few hassles, and sensitivity to the ecosystem are good medicine for curtailing cancer cells, bad quality of life, with lots of annoyances and insensitivity to ecosystem nurture and sustain cancer cells, like a dirty water puddle breeds mosquitoes. The instance of good Vedic sound (Sama Veda incantation) decreasing malignant cell growth was mentioned above. To the contrary, in the case of hard rock music the numbers turned positive in the wrong way as shown in Table 9 below.

Table 9: Decrease /Increase in Malignant growth - Sound of Samaveda Chant VS Hard Rock Music

Tissue or Organ	Classification	Cell Line	Sama Veda	Hard Rock
Brain	Malignant Glioma	U251-MG	-25.3	22.1
Breast	Adenocarcinoma	MCF7	-16.9	26.9
Colon	Adenocarcinoma	HT29	-19.9	14.1
Lung	Carcinoma	A549	-22.4	6.1
Skin	Malignant Melanoma	RPMI 7951	-12.4	Only one Experiment
Skin	Normal	NHDF	-13.9	10.2

Source: Adapted by author from Tables 13.1 and 13.2, Sharma H et al. Dynamic DNA

Patient's Resolve or Sankalpa Essential for Success

Yoga helps to look at an individual as a single energy field that can sustain a focused assault on unhealthy cells. The collective immune domain is summoned. This has a much better probability of success than just the micro quantifiable deductive approach. Healthy humans lack nothing in their immune defense system. Synergy comes into play in a big way. This approach to cancer treatment calls for resoluteness or "sankalpa" on the part of the patients who should not conjure up any inadequacy in their immune structure. A combined thrust of the immune system, energetic body and strongly willed mind, such a thrust constituting the sankalpa against cancer cells, can overpower them. Mental resolve helps substantially in buttressing the defense. A dogged faith in the capabilities of the inner defense structure to face the cancer challenge may help overpower the life-threatening cancer cells. *(Also see Chapter on Yoga and the Lymphatic System)*

In YA ambience, less is more. There is virtue in austerity and under-treatment rather than the other way around. Austerity invokes more rigor in the whole system which transmutes into a more holistic system. Even genes can be subjected to down- or upregulation, as needed, through simple method of guided meditation by the patient. Further discussion confirms the awesome potency of the immune system together with homeostasis that helps maintain the dynamic equilibrium in biological systems.

Yoga and meditation that affect analogous genes provide beneficial effects. Surprisingly, both during treatment and follow up periods, direct gene based depiction show little overlap in differently expressed genes. Cellular processes are regulated by consensus DNA sequences. Five protein complexes bind to these DNA sequences. The transcription factors that create the protein complexes constitute the nuclear factor kappa-light chain enhancer of activated B cells (NF-kB). The beneficial effects are: 1) Relaxation Response (RR) modified up-regulation of mitochondrial energy production by means of up regulation of ATPase and insulin function. 2) RR blunts down inflammation by down-regulating up- and downstream molecules of NF-kB molecules. NF-kB and other pro-inflammatory cytokines are the key molecules for ascribing beneficial effects of meditation. This is inferred from out of 21 meta-analysis studies. Big Data analysis of cancers and multiple myeloma bring out that RR effectively down regulates NF-kB associated with progression and resistance of multiple cancers.

There is emphasis today on the need to trust team communications which would make up for deficiencies if any in individual modality. [116] One conviction was that yoga helps in distress tolerance. It is successful in invoking the relaxation response so essential for cancer patients. The patient should make an educated guess in this respect and this could be helped by trying out a trial baseline eligibility for a potpourri of yoga and exercise protocols. At times the sick needlessly feel inadequate one way or other, such as for instance that their immune system is not strong enough to overwhelm cancer cells. This diffidence arises out of unawareness of the capabilities of the immune system or homeostasis or taking the body's defense too lightly.

YI Reduces Hospital Stay

Yoga intervention for wound healing and post-operative rehabilitation in the case of early operable breast cancer patients has been found to be significantly beneficial according to a randomized control trial of 2008[117]. This conclusion comes from a study with 69 patients, 33 in the yoga group and 36 in the control group, contributing data to statistical analysis. The patients' parameters were gathered at baseline prior to surgery and four weeks later. Duration of hospital stay, drain retention and time of suture removal besides post-operative complications were taken note of. Blood samples were collected to examine plasma cytokines—soluble Interleukin (IL)-2 receptor (IL-2R), tumor necrosis factor (TNF)-alpha and interferon (IFN)-gamma. Analysis showed significant decrease in duration of hospital stay (P = 0.003), days of drain retention (P = 0.001) and days of suture removal for the yoga group. The same group also showed a significant decrease in plasma TNF alpha levels following surgery (P < 0.001). The data was stable enough to have predictive value as per regression analysis of post-operative outcomes such as duration of hospital stay and TNF alpha levels.

YI and Prostrate Cancer

A 2013-14 clinical study brought out the effects of YI in prostate cancer. 15 patients (59 percent) were evaluable. Fatigue scores increased up to Week 4, and then scores improved in the course of the treatment (p = 0.008). Improvements in erectile deficiency, urinary incontinence (UI) and general QoL scores remained "reassuringly stable." The study concluded that a structured YI such as twice-weekly classes is feasible for prostate cancer patients undergoing 6-9 week outpatient radiotherapy. The study also reported promising results with stable scores for fatigue, sexual health, UI, and general QoL.[118]

Another 2019 study assessed YI in the clinical setting.[119] It dealt with women with cancer. In much of this assessment the holistic orientation dominated, such as inducing the relaxation response, bringing about a modicum of calmness to an otherwise disturbed mind, disturbed by a jumbo negative happening like cancer. In this setting, YI was supposed to have nothing direct to do with cancer, per se. Not surprising is the emphasis on hard-wiring of social connections as an imperative for reducing the symptoms of fatigue and negative emotions. The study reviewed randomized controlled trials (RCTs) of yoga in a research stream continuum (N = 29; n = 13 during treatment, n = 12 post-treatment, and n = 4 with mixed samples). Both during and after treatment, YI improved overall quality of life (QOL), with improvements in subdomains of QOL which varied across studies. Cancer-related fatigue was the most measured outcome among the RCTs. They all reported improvements in fatigue both during and after treatment. Results also suggested that yoga can improve stress/distress during treatment and post-treatment disturbances in sleep and cognition. Several RCTs provided evidence that yoga may improve biomarkers of stress, inflammation, and immune function. Outcomes with limited or mixed findings (eg, anxiety, depression, pain, cancer-specific symptoms, such as lymphedema) and positive psychological outcomes (such as benefit-finding and life satisfaction) warrant further study. Important future directions offered by oncologists for yoga research include: enrolling participants with cancer types other than breast, standardizing self-report assessments, increasing the use of active control groups and objective measures, and addressing the heterogeneity of yoga interventions, which vary in type, key components: movement, meditation, breathing, dose, and delivery mode and others.

Insightful are the results of 15-minute oncology massages to breast cancer patients during chemo in the infusion suites. The tests measured factors like nausea, anxiety, fatigue and pain decreased significantly. In another case of (Iyengar) yoga practice comparative results for the yoga group and the control group showed significant declines for yoga group in Brief Fatigue Inventory (BFI) Global score, BFI impact, BFI severity, and International Prostate Symptom Score (IPSS). The same study showed increases for the yoga group in FWB score, Functional Analysis of Cancer Therapy (FACT), Social Well-Being (SWB) and Sexual Health Inventory for Men (SHIM) scores.

For wider acceptance, yoga modality has been assessing YI in the clinical setting. One such assessment by Danhauer et al[120] refers to women with cancer. In much of this assessment the holistic orientation dominates, such as inducing the relaxation response, bringing about a modicum of calmness to an otherwise disturbed mind, disturbed by a mega-negative happening like cancer.

Hard-wiring of social connections would ameliorate patient wellness. The summary results from the 2019 study were that there were significant improvements for depression, negative effect, and health-related quality of life besides reduction in fatigue. In an earlier non-randomized pilot study of yoga for women with ovarian and breast cancer it was found there were significant improvements for depression, negative effect, anxiety, and QoL. The participants in the yoga program liked the new knowledge to use body-mind together, learning the relaxation techniques, relaxed peaceful feeling after yoga class, using breathing skills during MRI and the like. The study was not powered to detail group differences. However the decline in QoL for the yoga group was minimal. There were similar yoga choices for colorectal cancer patients and women with gynecologic surgery for malignancy. In general yoga skills in cancer cases helped with pain management. The strongest support from yoga was in alleviating anxiety, distress and mood. Moderate support was felt in sleep, fatigue and QoL.

The preliminary yoga support was in managing side effects, cognitive functions and spiritual wellbeing. The Table of outcomes of Randomized Control Trials is a useful reference to clinicians.[121] It was a good idea to offer a choice between cognitive behavioral therapy and yoga skills training, and build that choice into the design of clinical trials.

Overall it is agreed that there is sufficient evidence underpinning the benefits of yoga for those undergoing cancer treatment, both before, during and after moving into medical survivorship. Multiple level improvements in QoL are reported and evidenced, together with improvements in cancer-specific symptoms, physiological and mental functions and psychological outcomes. Improvements are also found in biomarkers such as stress hormone regulation, immune functions, and inflammatory markers. Cost-effectiveness was one of the other plus factors. It was suggested that yoga should be made available as part of standard cancer care. The outcomes have invariably been better for patients going into yoga more often. No adverse effects were reported due to yoga exercises, except rare case of muscle soreness.

Effect of yoga in palliative care and symptom management was the topic of a paper showing the results of a clinical yoga program on mood states, quality of life, and toxicity in breast cancer patients receiving conventional treatment.[122] This was a randomized control trial. There were significant results such as decrease in depression and distress in the yoga therapy group compared to the control group though both had similar baseline scores. The improvement in overall quality of life was by about 30 points compared to control group, proving that yoga as a psychotherapeutic intervention has considerable value for those cancer patients undergoing conventional treatment with improvements in psychological outcomes, reduction in symptom clusters and toxicity (p-value: <0.01). Some of the basics in health matters which are ignored or taken for granted, are relaxation poses, and breathing. Most persons are into inefficient breathing and thereby are not helping blood deliver oxygen to the trillions of cells in the body. Complementary medicine is often based on ancient practice. It has done successfully in clinical trials and otherwise proved itself highly efficacious, and is now on the rise, and on the map of healing systems. Cochrane Reviews are coming up with favorable appraisals of Ayurveda-Yoga notwithstanding the faulting of clinical studies for methodological inadequacies.[123, 124]

In the case of women with a diagnosis of breast cancer, under Cochrane Reviews, yoga therapy is recommended.[125] This is a meta-analysis of 17 studies under the Cochrane Database Systemic Review looking into the use of yoga as complementary therapy for breast cancer patients. 17 'moderate quality' studies compared yoga therapy and no therapy as control. The comparison found that

a) yoga improved health-related quality of life (HRQoL): pooled SMD 0.22, 95% CI 0.04 to 0.40; 10 studies, 675 participants;

b) Reduced fatigue (pooled SMD -0.48, 95% CI -0.75 to -0.20; 11 studies, 883 participants); and

c) Reduced sleep disturbances in the short term (pooled SMD -0.25, 95% CI -0.40 to -0.09; six studies, 657 participants).

However, the funnel plot for HRQoL was asymmetrical which meant that the inquiry results could be contaminated by publication bias and they did not favor any therapy. The funnel plot for fatigue was roughly symmetrical, meaning low risk of publication bias. Yoga did not appear to reduce depression in the case of some studies and the study also showed just the contrarian results of less depression (pooled SMD -0.13, 95% CI -0.31 to 0.05; seven studies, 496 participants; low-quality evidence; or anxiety (pooled SMD -0.53, 95% CI -1.10 to 0.04; six studies, 346 participants; very low-quality evidence. The overall conclusions by the authors of the study were that there was moderate-quality evidence recommending yoga as a supportive intervention for improving health-related quality of life and reducing fatigue, sleep disturbances, reducing depression, anxiety and fatigue, when compared with other psychosocial/educational interventions. The study also hinted that yoga might be as effective as other exercise interventions and might be used as an alternative to other exercises. It is not known the basis for this last suggestion, definitely it does not imply other exercises ameliorate fatigue, anxiety, depression or improve HRQoL. Besides serving as a supportive intervention in regard to HRQoL and fatigue, it would also be effective as an aerobic or cardiovascular exercise.

One of the earliest studies looked into the anxiolytic effects of yoga program and supportive therapy for breast cancer outpatients undergoing conventional treatment.[126] Out of a total sample of 98 stage II and III breast cancer outpatients, 45 patients were assigned to receive yoga therapy and 53 were to receive supportive therapy prior to surgery. However, only those who underwent surgery followed by adjuvant radiotherapy and six cycles of chemotherapy were picked for analysis. 18 of these were in the yoga therapy group and 20 in control group. Yoga intervention consisted of 60 minutes of yoga sessions whereas the control group had routine care of supportive therapy during hospital visits. The Spielbergers State Trait Anxiety Inventory and Symptom Checklist was used for assessments at baseline, after surgery, before, during and after radiotherapy and chemotherapy. General Linear Model (GLM) repeated measures ANOVA was employed to show in the yoga group a decrease in self-reported anxiety (p < 0.001) as well as trait anxiety (p = 0.005) as compared to controls. During conventional treatment intervals the results showed positive correlation between anxiety states and traits with symptom severity and distress. Yoga therapy is effective in reducing treatment-related symptoms and anxiety in breast cancer outpatients.

In order to improve the quality of life of cancer patients, the Institute of Medicine (IOM) has recommended that standard palliative care for them should include their psychosocial needs. The main complication here is that a variety of such psychosocial techniques are in use and they are not comparable. They range from cognitive behavioral stress management, and several speaking therapies to meditation, Qui Gong, yoga, individual expressive writing, and a variety of relaxation therapies. Just the global outcomes of these exercises may be comparable, like for instance survival rates and extent of health care utilization, but that may not be acceptable from a scientific point of view in terms of clinical tests, repeatability and dosage of the therapies. These issues are addressed in a 2013 study with psychosocial needs of mostly breast cancer patients under a broad psychoneuroimmunology umbrella.[127] The study included 24 clinical studies that had neuroendocrine-immune biomarkers as health outcomes. Two yoga-related clinical studies have been included in this work: those of Vadiraja HS et al[128] and Rao RM[129] et al. A diversity of methods or techniques was included in this study to evaluate the comparative outcomes of such techniques on PNI. Much care went into the study, and yet the diversity of interventions were such that the task of comparing even PNI cognitive-behavioral or complementary medical outcomes was rendered virtually futile.

Yoga in Post Cancer Survival

Yoga intervention for promoting survival in post-cancer life is being increasingly discussed. See for instance the 2019 study: The Impact of Yoga on Fatigue in Cancer Survivorship: A Meta-Analysis.[130] 29 studies made the grade for inclusion in this study and the total sample size was 1828 patients. Effect sizes (Hedge's g) were computed for fatigue, depression, and QoL. Statistically significant decrease in fatigue was noted: (g = 0.45, P = .013). The type of yoga was also a significant moderator of this relationship (P = 0.02). Yoga also was associated with decrease in depression, (g = 0.72, P = .007) but was not associated with statistically significant changes in quality of life (P = .48). The relationship between yoga and depression was conditioned by session length (P = 0.004.) When the comparator group was a waitlist or usual care group rather than when the control group was another active treatment group, the effect of yoga on fatigue and depression was larger. It was concluded that yoga may be advantageous as a component of treatment for both fatigue and depression in cancer survivors.

Some 1.8 million new cancer cases are estimated for 2020 and the number of projected cancer deaths are 606,520 which is about 33 percent of the new cases. The number of long term cancer survivors is increasing sizably. In 2016 there were 15.5 million persons classified as survivors, defined by the National Cancer Institute "as one who remains alive and continues to function during and after overcoming a serious hardship of life-threatening disease." A person is considered a survivor from the time of cancer diagnosis until the end of life. Survivors now constitute about 5% of the American population. And this is expected to go up with the increase in the number of survivors to 26.1 million in 2040.

The very diagnosis of cancer for many persons can be traumatic causing much distress and physical and psychosocial changes including free floating anxiety, fatigue, functional limitations, pain, cognitive and psychological issues. 90% of those undergoing radiation and chemotherapy experience CRF or cancer related fatigue. CRF continues during survivorship for many. There is also a link between CRF and depression, and inflammation and CRF. The levels of circulating markers of cytokine activity and elevated serum levels are both proinflammatory and could persist up to five years after diagnosis. In order to address the fatigue problem, holistic mind-body interventions, in particular yoga, are being looked into more frequently. Yoga includes physical and breathing exercises, the yoga package, together with meditation. According to the National Center for Complementary and Integrative Health, yoga is recommended to treat medical conditions such as cancer.

African American Women Study

The most diagnosed cancer amongst African-American Women is breast cancer. A-A Women are not known to engage in yoga as much as other ethnic communities. This 2018 pilot study[131] explored the feasibility of an 8-week restorative yoga program for African American breast cancer survivors (AA BCS) with respect to three criteria: a) How much better were the health outcomes in the restorative yoga (RY) group compared to wait list control group b) Was there adherence to RY program and c) What was the participant satisfaction assessment? 33 AA BCS were randomly assigned to either RY group (n = 18) or the control group (n = 15). Yoga classes met once a week for 8 weeks. Pre and post-tests were done at 0 and 8 weeks. The results were that the depression scores were significantly lower in the yoga group at M = 4.78, SD = 3.56, while in the wait list control group the scores were M = 6.91, SD = 5.86. There were no significant group differences in sleep quality, fatigue or perceived stress. Average rating of the yoga program was "very useful." While more exploration with larger samples are needed, there was clear evidence of decline in depression in AA BCS yoga group.

Yoga and Lymph Node Throat Cancer

What may be of interest to persons with cancer-related health problems is that yoga has successfully evolved from a mere exercise system into a fully-fledged treatment modality in its own right. It is getting institutionalized. It has emerged as an exposition of alround wellness. There are two aspects to modern yoga practice: first, as a mainstream technique it is under-serving the populace and second, in the process of diffusion and common practice, it is not been conforming to authentic yoga. As such there is concern as regards treatment employing yoga techniques and secondly its survival in terms of principles and practice of yoga in health care. Inter alia, yoga also helps with fasciae tissues that enclose muscles and separate them from internal organs. These matters about true yoga practices for intervention in cancer or other health problems can be resolved by recruiting certified and experienced yoga trainers.

There is the interesting case of metastatic cancer cells in the lymph nodes of Dr. Timothy McCall's his own neck and his visit to an Ayurvedic institution in Kerala, India. (See earlier references Table 7 and other pages) This was not as much for a cure, as for feeling more 'rested and balanced' before undergoing heavy-duty treatment such as chemo radiation. But after Ayurveda therapy the tonsil in his throat looked more pinkish healthy, and the lymph nodes shrunk, the size of the tumors slightly decreasing. After chemo radiation, McCall had a "complete clinical response," meaning lack of any evidence of cancer cells in his mouth or lymph nodes. Ayurvedic treatment prior to the heavy duty treatment made his body "hardier." This is the path of holism. When it comes to treatment of cancer per se, yoga has proved itself more holistic, moving more into the mind-body environment culture.

Yoga Heals Different Ways

Yoga looks into various imbalances and channels human effort towards ushering in the realm of para-sympathetic system. Yoga modality also tailors the treatment to the needs of the patient and his/her level of fitness. It includes breath and then involves the psychological aspects. There is left-side domination of yoga emphasizing mindfulness and also core strength which could serve as a prophylactic for osteoporosis. It is possible that some of the exercises could elicit the placebo effect, which by itself is not a fault. McCall lists 45 ways yoga heals. Just for illustration, it increases flexibility, strengthens muscles, improves balance and posture, improves lung function, slows and deepens breathing, uses imagery to effect change in body and relieve pain, lowers need for medication, leads to healthier habits, and encourages patient's own involvement in healing. He also mentions the popular vernacular axiom in India of the three health choices all people have in life: *yogi, bhogi* (one who is pleasure-oriented) and *rogi* (or the sick due to indulgences.)

Evidence shows that a) Yoga improves sleep, psychological well-being, Quality of Life, and possibly immune function in cancer patients, both during and after treatment. b) Yoga can improve risk factors or reduce probability of disease, something useful to cancer patients. c) Yoga therapy does not conform to the standardized sequences used in medical studies d) Yoga therapy that is tailored to individual needs are more effective than standard protocols e) Future studies should incorporate these suggestions. f) A wider number of cancer patients should be administered yoga interventions, now that benefits of such interventions as well as the low costs are confirmed. Yoga promotes wellness in a micro sense of personal wellness and second, in a macro way by promoting social harmony.

Yoga and Genomic Instability

Yoga-Ayurveda has the original lifestyle medicine. The Yoga Sutras advise "Avoid misery before they arise." The Bhagavad Gita exhorts "yuktahara viharasya ....." Be mindful of what diet and indulgences you have. Charaka Samhita states that there are two kinds of physicians: the superior ones that promote prana (life breath) and destroy roga (disease) and the inferior ones that pursue roga and destroy prana..." The human body is not a structure, but a process. It is an information and energy field. Evidence shows that genes have deterministic genetic codes, but as owner of the body, and with yoga expertise one can turn them on or off. The telomeres can be lengthened through yoga and good quality of life. This is true of brain structure and its wiring. Our relationship with time can be changed. We can transform and reinvent ourselves. Cancer hazards follow when there is disdain for health norms like being as close to nature as possible, consuming appropriate nutrition, resting as nature intended and related issues. American Cancer Society itself states that 90% of cancers are of environmental origin, with toxic chemical exposure, poor diet, drugs, radiation, stress and negative emotions contributing to genomic instability. According to the EPA our homes are 5 to 7 times more toxic than toxic waste dumps. 287 chemicals are found in new born babies according to the Environmental Working Group 2005. Some 400 cosmetic products are unsafe and some of the ingredients in them are banned in many countries. Averages of 100 pharmaceutical medicines are found in significant quantities in public drinking water.[132]

Carcinogenic Night Shift

The night shift for ladies in particular is labelled by WHO as the carcinogenic shift accounting for 19 percent of all cancers, 41% of skin cancer, 32% of breast cancer and 18% of GI cancer. The night shift is considered by many also as the graveyard shift in view of the heightened risk of common cancers especially among women. One large meta-analysis by researchers pulled together 61 research articles, involved 114,628 cases and 3,909,152 patients from Europe, N. America, Asia and Australia. Both the fixed effects model as well as the random effects model were employed.[133] To figure possible sources of heterogeneity, subgroup analyses and meta-regression analyses about breast cancer were conducted. A dose-response analysis was undertaken to estimate in quantitative terms the cumulative effect of night shift work on the risk of breast cancer.

The dose-response analysis revealed a positive correlation between long-term night shift work and risks of breast cancer [OR ¼ 1.316; 95% confidence interval (CI), 1.196–1.448], digestive system (OR ¼ 1.177; 95% CI, 1.065– 1.301), and skin cancer (OR ¼ 1.408; 95% CI, 1.024–1.934). What was egregious was that for every five years of night shift work, the risk of breast cancer in women increased by 3.3% (OR ¼ 1.033; 95% CI, 1.012– 1.056). In the case of night shift nurses, such night shift presented potential carcinogenic effect breast cancer (OR ¼ 1.577; 95% CI, 1.235–2.014), digestive system cancer (OR ¼ 1.350; 95% CI, 1.030–1.770), and lung cancer (OR ¼ 1.280; 95% CI, 1.070–1.531). This study more than confirmed the positive association between night shift work and common concerns in women. But when misclassifications and methodological errors in meta-analysis were pointed out this paper was retracted. Some 47 of the 61 remained in the study and results were the same.

Cancer risk for nurses doing night or swing shift increases by 58% as per sources mentioned above. Sleep itself is a miracle drug and its effect is underestimated at one's own peril. And so is fasting. The critical significance is brought out by the fact that there are peak times for numerous bodily functions.

For instance cortical catecholamine surge occurs in the morning between 6 and 9 AM. Plate adhesiveness and blood viscosity occurs around midday. Insulin is most produced between 5 and 6 PM. For wellness sake, eating, working, resting and other daily activities need to conform to the extent possible, to the peak time of metabolic activities. Ayurveda thus keeps an integrated 360 degree perspective on wellness that encases cure, maintenance and prevention.

Yoga Fosters Anti-Cancer Ecosystem

The silver Tsunami or the aging workforce as it is referred to, has an inexpensive option to cancer confrontation: consistent yoga practice, which has been upheld by research, especially for comfort in cancer treatment. Yoga is especially unmatched in the prevention of the emergence of the environment that entertains cancer. Cancer risk factors were modifiable. 30 to 50 percent of all cancers are preventable with healthy life styles and eschewing smoking, alcohol and sedentary habits. Conventional methods have become a "disease-based" approach to health care on account of conflicting challenges: a) cultural diversity in population that is being served, b) constraint imposed by the managed care system that regulates practice c) fears of litigation and d) boom in medical technology. In this disease-based ambience cancer treatment is also being verbalized. The medicines for treatment of cancer are too strong. Yoga health care can meet some of these challenges. Yoga can also be introduced in all work places. Earlier in the book, case studies have been mentioned of eminent physicians themselves cutting out panic and coming out clinically clean by making good use of ayurveda and yoga.

Till recently there was stigma attached to cancer like in the case of leprosy, making it more difficult to cure cancer elated issues. Stress causes some haplessness. It weakens critical parts of the brain and that makes one vulnerable. There are five pillars propping up integrated treatment of cancer and palliative care: 1) Recognize it as a problem 2) Take into account the cognition issues with cancer 3) Promote awareness of it 4) Discuss the not-always terminal risk 5) Don't underestimate the magnitude of the problem. Yoga's out-of-the-box solution capability should not be neglected.

Which Brain Wave to Invoke?

If the goal is to induce relaxation then it would be judicious to optimize factors that would elicit alpha waves if the yoga option is not available. If light meditation ambience is needed theta waves may be induced. Generation of extreme brain waves such as Delta (speed 0.5 – 40.0 Hertz cycles per second and Gamma 40 -100 Hertz) need to be minimized to avoid mental health issues. Each one of the waves has a specific purpose and function. Thus after a stress causing event Delta waves recorded in the frontal cortex enable osteoblast in which a cell secrets a matrix for bone formation. Mention of osteoblast in medical literature has increased dramatically in recent decades. These remedies apparently obfuscate issues when yoga can help generate the much-required Alpha waves (7.5 – 14 Hertz) so much more naturally through breathing exercises and relaxation poses. When the yoga option is very much available on tap, it is a slight to yoga to treat tension and stress other than non-pharmacologically. Meditation also has had proven success in reducing tension. Yoga was successful in 5 out of 7 cases.

Conclusion

In the transformation to integrated medicine it is essential that health care plays a role in diversification of modalities of treatment in the interest of best practices. Most often circumspection is called for in ayurveda or yoga intervention and every step needs documentation. This will come in handy in several ways including as a cure for a given condition. In carefully documented investigations it is possible to have Eureka moments, i.e., by happenstance coming across an effective remedy for a contentious cancer condition, besides deliberately leading to a successful solution to a medical condition.

Enough evidence has been adduced here of the effectiveness of YI at all stages of cancer especially when compared to control or routine therapy. While further research is definitely continuing to explore all aspects of YI, there is already adequate justification on the basis of available evidence to press on with yoga modality along with life style changes from ayurveda. If there is discomfort in taking to yoga-ayurveda ways despite the evidence, it is a straightforward case of one more illustration for the theory of cognitive discord as spoken of by Brehm et al.[134]

Chapter 12

Yoga and Asthma

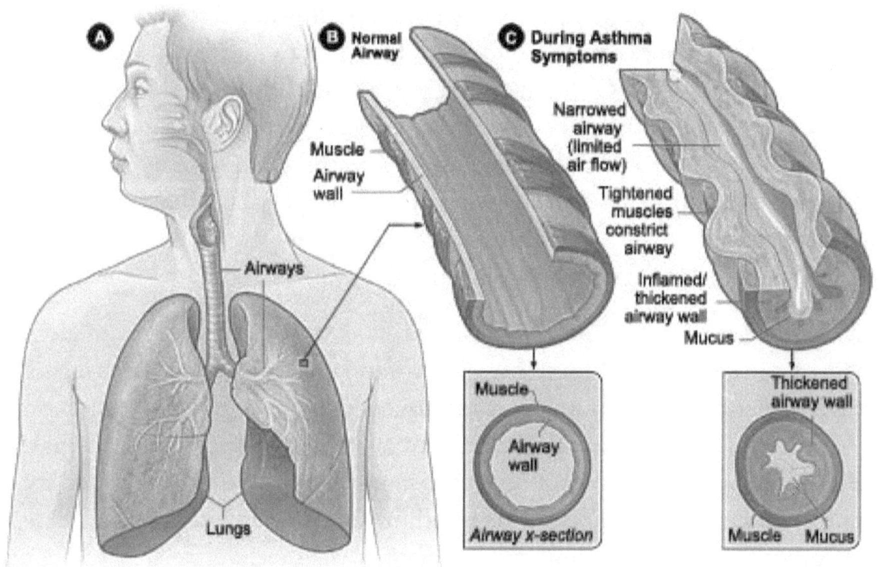

Fig 12: The Lungs and Airways

Source: U.S. Department of Health Services • National Institutes of Health

Yogic breathing and exercises are a prophylactic as well as a cure for most respiration-based illness like asthma, bronchitis, COPD, COVID, emphysema lung cancer, pneumonia and so forth. About 25 million persons in America and over a 100 million in India suffer from Asthma. Emergency Room visits due to asthmatic attacks are not uncommon, some two million of them in America per year. Asthma or bronchial asthma is a respiratory disease and is caused by the inflammation and narrowing of the airways to and from the lungs as shown in Fig.12-A, B and C. Pollen dust, pollution, smoke and even plain tension could cause inflammation. If not taken care of, asthma could lead to hypoxia or the lack of oxygen in blood which could affect brain function, as well as other parts of the body, overall severely sickening a person, and knocking out such a person's productivity and efficiency. More serious problems like heart attacks and stroke would be just waiting outside the door. When a person is having an asthmatic attack or spasm, swelling occurs inside the air passage, the muscles constrict and normal inhalation and exhalation is restricted. The breathing process becomes dysfunctional for the body.

It is easy to identify asthma sufferers. Besides having an inhaler, the asthma person feels a tightening or constriction of the airways and occasionally some chest pain too. They find it difficult to breathe due to narrowing of the bronchial tubes. Peak Flow meters measure this by way of lung function. Breaths are short, like that of a dog or a baby. Coughing is not uncommon. Mucus could be worsening the problem by choking up or obstructing whatever little air space is available in the airways. The wheezing is often audible. Breathing is labored. The wheezing and labored breathing is also known as dyspnea. They may have problems in speaking too and otherwise remain ruffled. Asthmatic persons find it not easy to fall asleep due to issues with breathing and the wheezing buzz.

Asthma can be occasional or persistent, mild or severe with combinations of these characteristics. The things that trigger asthma are varied from pollen dust, dog or pet hair and dander, ethnic food and flavors in food, smoking, psychosomatic reasons including anxieties, medicines and even exercise. Yoga helps to make it easier to breathe with breathing exercise, more by way of a prophylactic, not to underestimate curative function of breathing and other yoga exercises. One of the earliest controlled clinical studies to apply yoga techniques for asthma was the 1985 study by Nagarathna and Nagendra.[135] It matched the control and yoga groups in terms of, *inter alia,* age, severity of asthma, weekly drug score and also Mean Peak Expiratory Flow Rate (PEFR) measured by a flow meter. The PEFR measures the speed of expiration and tells the degree of obstruction in bronchial airways.

Table 10: YI in Asthma

Details of Patients	Control Group	Yoga Group
No. of Patients	53	53
Men	38	38
Women	15	15
Mean Age Range	26-41 (9-47)	26-46 (9-47)

Details of Patients	Control Group	Yoga Group
Mean Severity Score	1-45 (0-3)	1-45 (0-3)
No. with Seasonal Asthma	33	33
No. with Perennial Asthma	20	20
Mean Weakly Attack Range	3-08 (0-7)	3-01 (0-7)
Mean Weekly Drug Score Range	10-26 (0-49)	6-22 (0-21)
Mean Peak Flow Rate/1 min Range	264-2 (60-580)	290-1 (80-690)

Source: Nagarathna R and Nagendra HR https://www.ncbi.nlm.nih.gov/pmc/articles/ PMC1417003/?page=2

The Yoga Group (YG) and the Control Group (CG) consisted of 53 patients each, with equal number of men and women in both the groups. The YG practiced integrated yoga exercises consisting of breathing exercises, suryanamaskar, yoga asanas, dhyana or meditation and a devotional session. YG was asked to practice treatment lessons for 65 minutes every day. The main features like drug intake and peak flow rate were then compared with of the CG which continued to take the usual drugs for asthma. The YG showed significant improvements on the drug score, number of asthma attacks, and importantly on the PEFR. The Student's paired t test for mean differences for values before and after a 54 month follow up of YG and CG patients showed significant fall in the number of asthma attacks and significant increase in the PEFR. (P-Value < 0.05 for asthma attacks and drug use, and < 0.03 for PEFR. See Table 10 above)

There are Cochrane Reviews of clinical research into Yoga Intervention for Asthma. There is a 2020 study, but there is an embargo on its release till 2021. Leaving this aside, the latest is a 2016 study by Yang et al. This is more in the form of a meta-analysis or summary of all previous studies with summary results.[136] The reviewers follow the Cochrane Review rules and come up with strictly conservative conclusions such as Yoga improves quality of life of practioners and asthma symptoms to some extent, and not with specifics.

YI in Allergic Rhinitis

Common cold and allergies can cause rhinitis which is an inflammation of the mucous membrane in the nose. A 2017 study by Chellaa Rajesh et al[137] examined the impact of yoga training to manage the symptoms of allergic rhinitis. 51 healthy volunteers were recruited along with 51 allergic rhinitis patients. The researchers measured the upper airway resistance using a rhinomanometer and the lower airway resistance was measured using a spirometer. Specific yoga asanas were practiced for three months and airway resistance tests were done again. Data was collected using quality-of-life questionnaires in Short form-12 (SF-12) and the Sino Nasal Outcome Test (SNOT). The results from the paired student t tests showed significant reduction of total nasal airway resistance at 150 Pa (pressure in atmosphere) and significant increase in Forced Vital Capacity (FVC) during the pre- and post-yoga practice period. Forced Expiratory Volume (FEV1) and percent Residual standard deviation (%RSD) too went up, but not significantly. There was significant improvement in the Physical component score (PCS) and Mental component score (MCS) of the SF-12 health survey questionnaire. The SNOT questionnaire score came down significantly. Among the 51 rhinitis patients the Total Nasal Airway Resistance went down significantly at 150 Pa and the FVC pre yoga and post yoga scores showed some increase that was not significant. FEV1 and% RSD significantly increased. These are significant findings about the impact of yoga practices for diseases of the bronchial air tubes or airways.

Yoga Breathing is not unique. However, it needs to spread because of ubiquitous prevalence of unnatural breathing mainly due to frenetic and feverish living styles. The average person's common breathing is alarmingly inefficient. This one reason alone could be the trigger for scores of illnesses, including cardio-vascular diseases, asthma, headaches, foul moods, anxieties, tension, stress, and that is saying a lot. Besides inefficient breathing there is also paradoxical breathing, something this author has witnessed in all age ranges from 5 to 90 years. (See Chapter 8 on Yoga and Common Sense.)

Yoga Helps Fuller Utilization of Lung Capacity

Total lung capacity of a healthy human is estimated 6000 milliliters, 3000 ml in each one of them. The left lung has two lobes and the right lung, three. And woefully, each normal breath a person breathes in, is about 250 or 300 ml or about ten percent of the capacity. Even a long drawn abdominal breath could have a maximum of 500 ml or about 16.7%. Deep abdominal (belly) breathing helps the brain cells and neurons receive more oxygen and thereby helps the person to keep the central nervous system bathe in oxygen and stay impervious to emotions. This is a coveted mental state, the reason for people undertaking meditation. This is also the first step in decision-making, especially those decisions that impact life on *terra firma*.

Several studies over the decades have proved that breathing exercises prescribed in yoga help rediscover lung capacity. One such study of the effect of yoga breathing exercise undertaken by 18 women soccer players confirmed that such breathing improved total lung capacity. The sample was divided into Group A and Group B with nine women in each. The first group served as the experimental group and practiced yogic breathing and the other (control group) didn't. The duration of the exercises for Group A was six weeks, practiced five days a week, and each breathing session lasted an hour. The control group B did not undertake any specific exercise in breathing, but went about with regular routine activities. The lung capacity was assessed with the help of a spirometer test. Pre- and Post-exercise scores were thus collected and a statistical dependent test, also known as paired sample t-test, and an Analysis of Covariance (ANCOVA) test were done. The conclusion of this study was that the yoga breathing exercises group had shown significantly improved total lung capacity. The control group had not shown any significant improvement in total lung capacity[138]

One of the case control studies on yogic breathing is from Lahore, Pakistan. This study was to check on the impact of Bhastrika, Pranayama and Humsa breathing techniques on heart rate (HR), systolic blood pressure (SBP), and peak expiratory flow rate (PEFR). The sample sizes were 100 for the treatment group and 50 for the control group. Physical characteristics (age, height, and weight) were recorded and medical history was obtained from both groups of subjects. The subjects' cardiorespiratory responses were assessed before and after the pranayama (Yogic breathing) session. Yogic breathing techniques were demonstrated and practiced for 1 hour by the Treatment Group under expert guidance. When the before and after data were analyzed in each group, the mean values for Heart Rate and Systolic BP in the treatment group were significantly decreased after the pranayama session while PEFR significantly increased. Yogic breathing improved the subjects' cardiorespiratory responses in the Treatment Group.[139]

Asthma is no more an uncommon ailment for millions of people. Yoga abhors any restraint on breathing because the main objective of yoga exercises is to facilitate the delivery of oxygen efficiently to the trillions of cells in the human body, and instantly reduce stress. For this purpose it lays much emphasis on exercises for perking up the respiratory system and the connected blood circulation.

Wheezing and the shortness of breath are, unfortunately, very stressful symptoms of someone with asthma. Until recently the conventional cure for asthma was medication, usually steroids taken through inhalers. This treatment dilates the air tubes and brings relief. However it only suppresses the symptoms, and does nothing to address and cure the underlying breathing problem. After recognizing the adverse effects on many patients, healthcare providers began seeking out alternative ways to treat asthma. Thus, the recommendation today is yoga breathing. In Britain 88 percent of asthma victims stated that they found a lasting remedy in yogic breathing. See Table 7, page 42. This author's own asthma students confirm this fact.

Most asthma patients do not belly breathe the way that healthy people do. Breathing is shallow and could be clavicular or thoracic. In clavicular breathing, a person's shoulder bones alone are moving up and down with inhalation and exhalation. Such thin breathing does not fill all the five compartments of the two lungs. Without a full breath the body cells are not getting the necessary amount of oxygen to keep them healthy. Thoracic breathing is also an insufficient form of breathing. Just inflating and deflating the ribcage while breathing is thoracic breathing. While it is better than clavicular, it is still not adequate for all metabolic functions.

Best Breathing Practices

The only kind of breathing that fills the available space in lungs is abdominal breathing. This natural form of breathing happens when the breath is inhaled fully, the diaphragm extending the stomach or inflating the abdominal area below the rib cage, and deflating the area on the exhale. Some shallow breathers even do paradoxical or reverse breathing, which could undernourish the blood of oxygen. When they inhale, their stomachs go in concave to the spine, rather than out; and when they exhale the stomach inflates convex to the spine! How much better they would feel if only they could be taught to breathe normally!

For people who wheeze and even those that have other respiratory issues like Corona Virus infection, there are excellent yoga breathing practices. Besides, the bellows or bhastrika, there is the *Nadishodhana,* or *nadi shuddha Pranayama* or single and alternate nostril breathing. There are others like Sheetali and Brahmari breathing. Besides curing asthma and breathing problems of that kind, for purposes of physical and mental fitness too, deep belly breathing is essential. Empirical research has brought out how breathing exercises enhance breathing capacity with much significance for oxygen delivery for the trillions of cells through enriched blood.

Several clinical studies over the decades have proved that exercises such as abdominal breathing help rediscover lung capacity and improve sports performance. As fresh air goes deeper into the lungs, there is more oxygenation of blood, helping deliver more of the life force (*pran* in *Sanskrit*). Runners at

University of Portsmouth who included breathing in their training improved their running times by 5 to 12%. Breathing exercises in the run up to sports event helped such participants stay calm, without anxiety, and helped increase speed, endurance and strength, giving an edge on the big day.[140]

Another clinical research looking into the effect of breathing exercise undertaken by 18 women soccer players confirmed that deep breathing improved total lung capacity utilization. This has been referred to on page 129.[141]

(Note to reader: How do we perform Nadishodana Pranayama? The steps are given below)

Nadishodhana Pranayama (NP) or single and alternate nostril breathing
1. Bend your middle and index fingers and using the ring finger and thumb make a clip. Clip both nostrils and block the inflow or outflow of breath.
2. Gently press your nostrils closed with your "clip" such that no air escapes.
3. Open the left nostril by loosening the finger on the left side of the nose and exhale as long as you can
4. Inhale through the same left nostril as deeply as you can, filling out the lungs.
5. Hold the breath, clipping both nostrils firmly, and curve your neck enough to press the chin to the chest below the Adam's apple (bump on the inside throat or larynx). Press the chin against chest. It will lock the air in, and also massage the thyroid and parathyroid organs under the neck and improves their health.
6. Hold the breath as long as you can without straining, then lift the neck, open the right nostril and slowly exhale, (the slower the better). If you have held the breath too long, you will be breathing out with a big puff! So don't strain to hold the breath longer than is comfortable.
7. Inhale slowly through the same right nostril and again: hold the breath, bend the neck forwards, and put the chin against the chest below the Adam's apple as before in step 5 above.
8. Hold the breath as long as possible and then: raise the head, open the left nostril and exhale as slowly as possible. This completes one round of *Nadishodhana Pranayama.*
Note: *NP can be done as often as possible and at any time of the day, leaving at least two hour gap before lunch/dinner. NP and bhastrika could be the best prophylactics against asthma.*

Chapter 13

Yoga and Diabetes

Diabetes, or *diabetes mellitus*, refers to disorders characterized by high glucose levels in blood and larger urine production. When diabetes is followed by lower secretion of vasopressin by the pituitary gland the disorder takes the name of diabetes insipidus, which is otherwise not related to diabetes. The main reason for high blood sugar is inadequate insulin generated by pancreas located in the abdominal (belly) cavity. Pancreas, according to some, are not an endocrine gland. It's but a collection of cells going by the name of *islets of Langerhans* which have the functionality of an endocrine gland, producing hormones such as insulin and glucagon. These hormones control blood sugar levels. And as hard luck would have it, the pituitary-hypothalamus system does not regulate the pancreatic function.

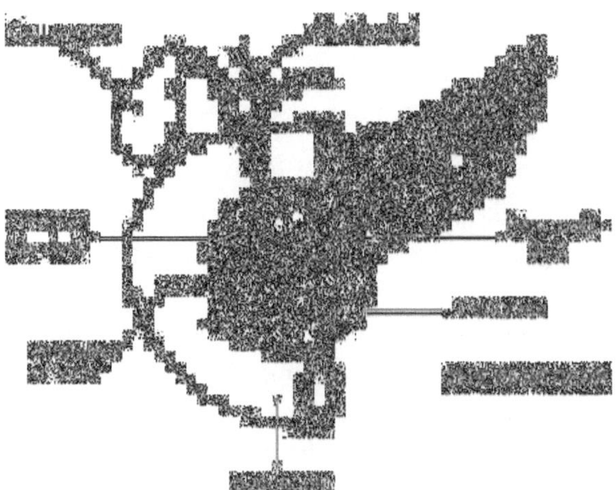

Fig.13: The Pancreas: *islets of Langerhans*

Source: Dept. of Work and Pensions, UK Govt.

Without insulin generated by the pancreas sugar cannot enter the body cells, nor can they burn (use up) sugar in blood to convert it into energy. Liver stores sugar.

Glucagon helps breakdown the sugar. When we exercise or when stressed out, glucose is secreted.

In Type 1 diabetes (also known as IDDM for Insulin Dependent Diabetes Mellitus), pancreatic cells are attacked by one's own immune cells by mistake. At times it is an inherited disorder and those suffering from it tend to have abnormal levels of antibodies (blood proteins). In Type 2 diabetes, (also known as NIDDM: Non-Insulin Dependent Diabetes Mellitus or adult onset diabetes mellitus) the pancreas produce insulin not adequate to the body requirement. At times the pancreas produces more insulin, but the fat and muscle cells in the body become insensitive to insulin. This is insulin resistance. Sugar and glucose in blood sugar get elevated as a result.

When pancreas cannot produce adequate insulin or when the body cannot utilize it, hyperglycemia, or raised blood sugar, occurs and it goes by the name of diabetes. According to the World Health Organization the number of people with diabetes, the 7th leading cause of death, went up from 108 million in 1980 to 422 million in 2014.[142] Global prevalence in ages 18 years and above went up from 4.7 to 8.5% of population during the same period. Between 2000 and 2016 premature mortality from diabetes increased by 5%. The number of deaths directly caused by diabetes is estimated at 1.6 million in 2016. 50% such deaths occur before the age of 70 years. With diabetes comes serious other health risk factors like macrovascular complications, atherosclerosis, cardiovascular disease, retinitis, diabetic neuropathy, renal disease, depression, dementia and associated complications.

That it occurs in such increasing numbers because of poor diet, lack of exercise, leading to overweight and obesity, is a poor commentary on life styles even as personal income increases. Some patients and some in the medical establishment too, appear to be convinced that life styles like eating high cholesterol and sugary foods and beverages in large proportions, not moving the body much, are nonmodifiable factors! Not surprisingly the lines to get into hospitals and clinics for diabetes treatment are lengthening. Diabetes-related health care costs are bound to burgeon beyond the current 10% of total health care costs.

Commensurate and statistically sound evidence by way of both random and nonrandom controlled studies has been marshalled to support that yoga does benefit Diabetes Mellitus Type 2 (DMT_2) patients. Yoga practices help increase insulin output, makes the body take it in good measure, reduces blood sugar and otherwise reduces medication.

Table below is one such evidence which in terms of rigor and other criteria checks all the boxes. The 2016 research paper (Kim EI et al 2016)[143] speaks of a pandemic of DMT2 especially in the last three decades, say beginning in the 80s that has led to more than doubling of the number of DMT2 cases. The current number of diabetes sufferers is about 470 million and this is projected to go up to 522 million by 2030.

Recent published meta-analyses regarding effects of yoga on risk indices relevant to T2DM, in summarized form are presented below.

Table 11: Clinical Data of YI in T2DM

	NRCTs (*N*)	RCTs (*N*)	Total *N*	%
Participant characteristics				
Target population: adults with				
Type 2 diabetes only	12	12	24	96.00%
Unspecified diabetes	1	0	1	4.00%
One gender only specified	0	2	2	8.00%
Excluding those on DM meds				
Yes	2	0	2	8.00%
Not specified	0	1	1	4.00%
Excluding those with DM complications				
Yes	9	10	19	76.00%
No	1	1	2	8.00%
Not specified	3	1	4	16.00%
Age range in years				
≥18–26	0	3	3	12.00%
30/35–55/60/65	6	2	8	32.00%
40/45–55/60	3	2	5	20.00%
40/45–65/70/75	3	2	5	20.00%
50–70/>60 y	0	2	2	8.00%
Not specified	1	1	2	8.00%
Years since DM diagnosis				
≥0-1 year	0	2	2	8.00%
1/2 years	1	0	1	4.00%
2–5 years	0	1	1	4.00%
5–10 years	0	1	1	4.00%

	NRCTs (N)	RCTs (N)	Total N	%
0/1–10 years	7	1	8	32.00%
>15 years	0	2	2	8.00%
Not specified	5	5	10	40.00%
Sample size				
<25	0	2	2	8.00%
25–40	2	2	4	16.00%
41–60	4	4	8	32.00%
>60	7	4	11	44.00%
Location				
India	13	7	20	80.00%
UK	0	2	2	8.00%
Cuba	0	2	2	8.00%
Iran	0	1	1	4.00%
Year published				
2010–2014	7	7	14	56.00%
2005–2009	2	3	5	20.00%
2000–2004	3	1	4	16.00%
Prior to 2000	1	1	2	8.00%
Yoga intervention*				
Yoga-based program alone				
Including asanas	11	10	21	84.00%
Not including asanas	0	2	2	8.00%
Yoga combined with other interventions				
Including asanas	3	0	3	12.00%

	NRCTs (N)	RCTs (N)	Total N	%
Not including asanas	0	0	0	0.00%
Duration				
<8 weeks	6	1	7	28.00%
12 weeks/3 months	5	7	12	48.00%
4–6 months	2	2	4	16.00%
>6 months	0	2	2	8.00%
Frequency of practice¥				
<3x/week	0	1	1	4.30%
3x/week	1	3	4	17.40%

	NRCTs (*N*)	RCTs (*N*)	Total *N*	%
4-5x/week	2	1	3	13.00%
6-7x/week	8	7	15	65.20%
Program structure¥¥				
Classes only	9	7	16	69.60%
Classes combined with home practice	1	5	6	26.10%
Training session combined with home practice	1	0	1	4.30%
Comparison condition**				
Usual care/no treatment	11	8	19	76.00%
Attention control	0	1	1	4.00%
Active comparator	3	5	8	32.00%
>1 control	1	2	3	12.00%

*Including two yoga-based interventions tested within the same study [38]. ¥Practice frequency not specified in 2 NRCTs. ¥¥Information on program structure lacking in two NRCTs [39, 41]. **Numbers add up to more than 25, as 3 studies included more than one comparator.
Source: Kim EI et al 2016[144]

The 2016 study examined a number of controlled trials systematically and it concluded that yogic practices may promote significant betterments in indices such as glycemic control, lipid levels, and body composition that matter in the management of DM2. Some of the controlled trials which the 2016 study examined highlighted other benefits of YI: lower oxidative stress and BP, enhanced pulmonary and nervous system function, better mood, sleep and quality of life, and reduced medication in adults with DM2. It also listed heterogeneity of the studies that call for caution in interpreting results.

Yoga has numerous remedies for diabetes such as Halasana, Sarvangasana, Dhanurasana, Ardhmatsyendrasana, which impact the digestive organs including pancreas and liver. A holistic approach including nutrition and dietetics will yield the best results in managing diabetes, and in promoting insulin production. Digestive physiology also improves making it possible to have the maximum impact.

BKS Iyengar's *Light on Yoga* in Annexure II on Curative Asanas for Diseases lists many others including Akarna Dhnaurasana, Sirsasana, Uttanasana and others.

One of the 2014 studies was a parallel randomized controlled study to collect efficacy data on yoga intervention in diabetes. One of its limited objectives was to check if YI could rein in weight-related diabetes risk factors.[145] Accordingly, more than blood sugar level, the study focused on changes in BMI, waist circumference, fasting blood glucose, insulin, insulin resistance and so forth. The study was comprehensive in coverage and included changes in depression, anxiety, positive and negative affect and perceived stress. The study randomized 41 participants with elevated fasting blood glucose in Bangalore, India to either a yoga group (n = 21) or a walking control (n = 20). While the yoga group had to attend yoga classes and the control group was asked to walk 3-6 days per week for 8 weeks. The study was practicable in terms of recruitment, retention and adherence. The yoga group registered significantly greater reductions in weight, waist circumference, and BMI as compared to the control. The results are in Table 12 below:

Table 12: YI and Diabetes Risk Factors

Risk Factor	Yoga Group	Control	P-Value
Weight	-0.8 ± 2.1	1.4 ±3.6	0.02
Waist Circumstance	-4.2 ± 4.8	0.7±4.2	<0.01
BMI	-0.2 ± 0.8	0.6 ± 1.6	0.05
Fasting BG	No Significant Differences in both		
Postprandial BG	No Significant Differences in both		
Insulin Resistance	No Significant Differences in both		
Psychological Wellbeing	No Significant Differences in both		
Blood Pressure Systolic and Diastolic	Significant Reductions in both groups		
Total Cholesterol	Significant Reductions in both groups		
Anxiety, Depression, Negative affect	Significant Reductions in both groups		
Perceived Stress	Significant Reductions in both groups		

Source: McDermott KA et al [145]

The conclusion: YI has the promise of decreasing weight-related diabetes risk factors and improving psychological well-being.

Another 2013 Indian study[146] was able to point to significant effects of YI in diabetes. 100 DMT2 patients with dyslipidemia were randomized into a yoga group (YG) and a control group (CG). The YG practiced yoga for one hour daily along with oral hypoglycemic drugs for 3 months. The CG just took the the same drug. After 3 months, the YG had a reduction in total cholesterol, triglycerides, and LDL, and an increase in HDL. Details are in Tables 13 and 14. The Study concluded that yoga targets elevated lipid levels in diabetes patients.

Table 13 Comparison of pre-yoga and post-yoga values in experimental group.

Parameters *n* = 50	Pre-yoga (mean ± SD)	Post-yoga (mean ± SD)
WT(kg)	62.20 ± 4.45	59.60 ± 4.65*
BMI (kg/m²)	25.12 ± 1.54	23.59 ± 1.38
W/H ratio	0.94 + 0.07	0.89 + 0.07*
Total cholesterol (mg/dl)	244.86 ± 28.09	219.54 ± 32.02**
Triglycerides (mg/dl)	151.88 ± 43.08	130.11 ± 28.82*
LDL cholesterol (mg/dl)	144.74 ± 28.45	120.51 ± 34.31**
HDL cholesterol (mg/dl)	44.63 ± 9.35	47.15 ± 8.17

$*p < 0.05$, $**p < 0.01$.

Source: Shantakumari N. et al 2013

Table 14: Comparison of initial values of parameters and follow up values of the control group.

Parameters n = 50	Initial value (mean ± SD)	Follow up (mean ± SD)
WT (kg)	62.17 ± 4.67	63.03 ± 5.10*
BMI (kg/m²)	24.73 ± 1.87	25.03 ± 2.14
W/H ratio	0.93 + 0.07	0.91 + 0.05
Total cholesterol (mg/dl)	225.74 ± 37.60	235.23 ± 26.64
Triglycerides (mg/dl)	172.74 ± 52.55	197.91 ± 130.11
LDL cholesterol (mg/dl)	126.11 ± 30.41	126.60 ± 22.84
HDL cholesterol (mg/dl)	44.23 ± 5.21	43.13 ± 12.33

$*p < 0.05$.

Source: Shantakumari N. et al 2013

As noted above a 2016 study systematically examined a number of controlled studies and concluded that there significant improvements in glycemic control, lipid levels, and in body composition of much relevance in DM2 management.[147]

In a 2018 review of studies of YI in diabetes a complete list of practices from the yoga package such as asanas, mudras, kriyas, bandhas and breathing, besides ideal diet for such a condition has been given in detail.[148] One of the most novel suggestions of this study was that psychoneuro-endocrine and immune mechanisms have holistic effects in diabetes control. This is the DNA of yogic practice: to work in a comprehensive way so that the root-causes of any particular illness can be addressed, not just the symptoms. For instance, parasympathetic activation and stress management, so much an integral part of yoga practice, would perk up metabolic and psychological profiles of diabetic patients, increase their insulin sensitivity, glucose tolerance as well as lipid metabolism. Along with DM2, if there are other comorbidities, YI are likely to take care of them too in the process of reduction of blood glucose levels. In view of this collateral progress, the review concluded that there could be other significant positive clinical outcomes from YI.

While yoga practices from the yoga package are critical for blood sugar control, diet cannot be ignored. There needs to be a modicum of limits on fat, sugar and carb inputs from fruit juices, soda, cookies, hot dogs, cheese, and their like. Further Yoga-Ayurveda would also urge that juices of vegetables like bitter gourd, neem leaves, kale, broccoli, radishes, and their like be consumed in prescribed doses so that they may provide a natural insulin substitute.

Chapter 14

Yoga and Backache

Every time we sit, stand, walk, lift objects or twist the lumbar area the spine is at work. Without the spine the back would collapse into the ribcage pressuring the lungs and the heart. Standing erect and walking would be impossible. The human body would always slouch, and either bend forward or backward, making it impossible to do even simple things. Equally important, the spine is the trunk-line for communications between the neurons in the brain and the billions of cells all over the body. When the spine is not in good health; our reflexes slow down, endangering us and others, such as for instance, when we are driving. Poor back health slows down all physical activity, making us inefficient in anything we do. An overwhelming majority of adults, some 80 percent, suffer from back aches.

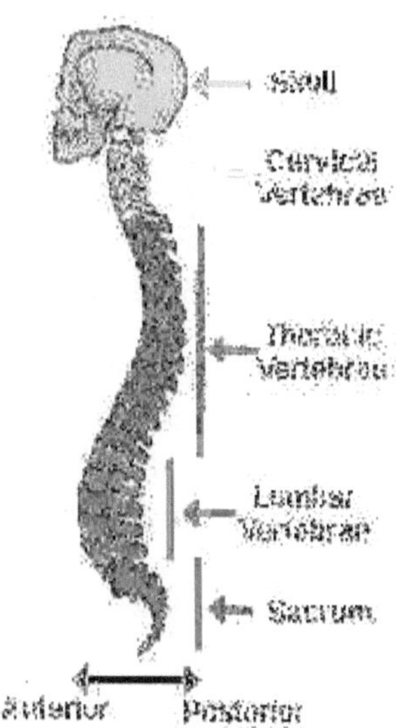

Fig 14: The Spine with Vertebrae

Source: faculty.washington.edu

It is therefore most important to prevent back aches caused by straining the back while lifting heavy objects the wrong way, or sitting in a wrong posture for a long time either at a work desk or while driving. Other activities that contribute to back aches are: slouching while sitting, sleeping on improper pillows and beds, and not doing back exercises regularly. Sitting with a slouch can hurt the spine and also stop proper breathing. Improper breathing leads to numerous physical and even mental issues.

Yoga and Back Pain

Back pain could be in the upper back in the shoulders, the cervical or clavicular area, the shoulder blades, the lumbar, sacrum or tailbone or any part of the spine. The reason for back pain could be several. As noted above, it could be caused by lifting heavy materials without caution. One can get a back ache just carrying an ill-fitting backpack. Many persons wake up with a back pain or a neck pain or both. There could be ergonomic causes for a spine-related or a sciatica problem.

Back pain is a common ailment not just for humans, but even for animals. About a quarter to a third of the human population could be suffering from back ache sometime or the other. In America about 10 per cent of the population or 33 million persons could be experiencing backache at any one time. There is a big loss of human productivity and loss of millions of man hours every year. Some 300 million days are lost to the economy and may be lot more in the informal business and charity sectors including in the unpaid household sector, like the services of a multipurpose mother. The American Chiropractic Association estimates the dollar cost of back ache at about $100 billion (2015) including cost of treatment and man hours lost.[149]

The recovery time from back ache depends upon the severity, cause of the ache, work culture and ergonomic reasons, age and life styles. Increasingly yogic exercises are being prescribed for back ache. This trend towards yoga modality for back ache will gain momentum in the coming years as its efficacy in complete resolution of the back ache problem, as compared to partial or momentary resolution by other modalities, especially the pharmacological means, comes to be known. Equally interesting, the cost to the person that has learnt the exercises for back ache is just the tuition fee of a couple of hundred dollars for the yoga exercises. The return on investment of this amount would be cost of treatment for backache every time one gets it. No other modality can be that effective and at the same time that easy on the pocket. If back ache sufferers take to yoga, it would impact the nation's health care costs significantly.

YI RCTs for Back Ache

A 2007 review of six RCTs found strong evidence for people with chronic low back pain (LBP) that unloaded movement facilitation exercises (techniques based on yoga asanas such as Bhujangasana and Svanasana) decreased pain and improved functionality as compared to no exercise.[150] The six studies included were classed as high quality with a mean quality assessment score of 7.7 out of a possible 10. The study included what is called a McKenzie Therapy (MT) which is probably modified Bhujangasana and Shavanasana. The therapy was developed by Robin McKenzie, New Zealand. As reported in the 2007 study:

- MT was found to be more effective than other exercise for short-term pain (SMD 0.38, 95% CI: 0.14, 0.61; 2 trials, n=289), but not short-term function (SMD 0.10, 95% CI: -0.20, 0.40; 2 trials, n=289).
- Yoga was more effective than education, self-care and no exercise for medium-term pain (SMD 0.92, 95% CI: 0.47, 1.37; 2 trials, n=88) and medium-term function (SMD 0.95, 95% CI: 0.50, 1.40; 2 trials, n=88).
- Yoga and MT together were more effective than other exercise for short-term pain (SMD 0.36, 95% CI: 0.15, 0.58; 3 trials n=336) and medium-term pain (SMD 0.39, 95% CI: 0.16, 0.61; 2 trials, n=309).
- Yoga + MT were more effective than education, self-care and no exercise for medium-term pain (SMD 0.53, 95% CI: 0.12, 0.94; 4 trials, n=251) and medium-term function (SMD 0.51, 95% CI: 0.00, 1.02; 4 trials, n=309).

The authors' conclusions were that compared to no exercise, yoga and yoga-based techniques such as Bhujangasana and Svanasana are effective for improving pain and functionality for people with non-specific chronic LBP.

There is considerable research into yoga intervention including random clinical trials for backache. One such is a 2016 study. It was an exhaustive survey of the literature on the topic. The study stated that "It is the most common cause of limited activity in people below the age of 45, is the second most frequent reason for visits to a physician, the third most common reason for surgery, and the fifth most common cause of hospital admission in the United States."[151] It started with an initial survey of 127 PubMed studies and then whittled it down to incontrovertible evidence studies of just 14. Most of the studies reviewed were ranked 2-4 under the Oxford Centre for Evidence Based Medicine 2011 Levels of Evidence criteria. The studies reported less pain, more energy, less symptoms of depression, better HR Quality of Life, reduced functional disability and so forth.

The yoga exercises were the familiar ones that students get to do in a yoga class. It included breathing and related relaxation exercises too. The mechanism by which yoga cures back ache was studied with reference to yoga's impact on biochemicals of the yoga person. They included serotonin, cortisol, dehydroepiandrosterone (DHEA), and brain derived neurotrophic factor (BDNF). One study included in the review looked at psychological factors that could impinge on pain abatement due to yoga. The beneficial effects of yoga were related to elevated serum BDNF levels and high serotonin levels.

One study (Lee et al) investigated the effect of yoga on pain, BDNF, and serotonin in premenopausal women with chronic low back pain.[152] The yoga group had decreased pain, increased BDNF and unchanged serotonin. The untreated control group had increased pain, decreased BDNF and decreased serotonin. Elevated serum BDNF levels and sustained serotonin levels were attributed to the yoga effect. There were no serious adverse events following yoga exercises and so yoga is considered safe. No doubt there were a few complaints attributed to taking to yoga for the first time, with tenderness in some part of the back or in arms and limbs. One person complained of migraine headache after the exercises and another reportedly went for Chiropractic help. These incidents were not severe, nor injurious and so could be due to not exercising caution either by the patient or the yoga instructor. Majority of the yoga participants appreciated the beneficial impact of yoga intervention.

The study noted that yoga intervention with its emphasis on both prevention and cure, fits in well with the emerging trend in America of shifting from treating patients with acute illness to those with chronic disease including trauma. The meditative and reflective influence of yoga would lend itself well for veterans especially for veterans with PTSD. The study concludes that the functional disability of back ache is well taken care of by YI which makes back ache less bothersome as an independent modality, and also especially in comparison with other traditional modalities. The overall conclusion was: "Yoga may have a positive effect on depression and other psychological co-morbidities, with maintenance of serum BDNF and serotonin levels. Yoga appears to be an effective and safe intervention for chronic low back pain."[153]

Before going for acupuncture, pills, hormones, pain relievers and even surgery, those suffering from back ache should first try simple yogic remedies. *A:sanas* that are highly recommended are the *svanasana* (dog pose) for lower back ache, and *bhujangasana* for the upper back pain, including for the neck and shoulders. Accurate and regular performance of these, or other *asanas* such as *shalabasana, dhanurasana, urdvadhanura:sana, sarvangasana, oustrasana* and several others, would not only prevent back ache but would also serve as effective and tested medicine for an existing problem. Ancient sages devised them after a sound understanding of the biomechanics of the spine. The remedial poses constitute a biomechanical-psycho-social cure to back aches.

Svanasana for lower back

Contraindications: Don't attempt if having respiratory problems, joint pain, slipped disk, high BP, weak spine and related issues

Method: Lie down on your stomach, face down, head resting on forehead.

- Keep palms flat on the floor near the chest, forearms hugging your torso
- Take a good breath, scrape your nose and chin on the floor in the same order, and slowly lift your head and toss head back as far as possible.
- Press your palms into the floor, lift the torso, and hips. Now the only two contact points with the floor are your palms and toes. The knee is above the floor. Slowly drag your torso forward, even while retaining the knee and palm contact with the floor.
- Drop the hip low and make the torso as vertical as possible without hurting; point your toes, and keep them together.
- Take deep breaths and stay in that posture as long as you can, say a minute or more.
- When you want to come out of the pose, slowly slide back, bring your torso down to the floor, scrape chin and nose, in that order and rest head on the forehead as in the starting posture.

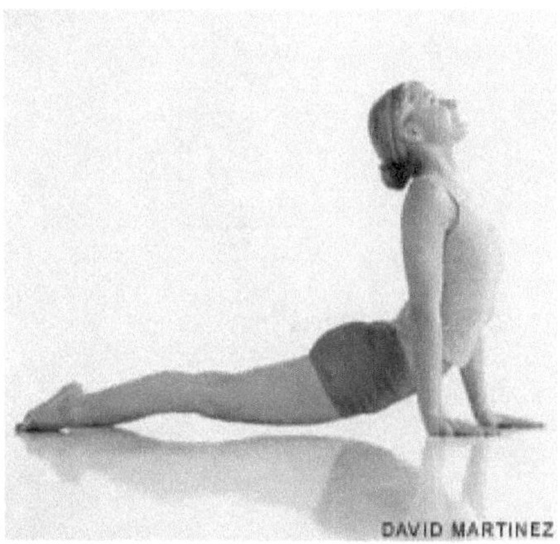

Svanasana

Bhujangasana **for Upper Back**

Contraindications: Don't do any asanas if you have joint pain, slipped disk, high BP, spinal problems or aches.

Method: The starting posture is the same as in *Sva:na:sana*.

- After taking a good breath, scrape the chin and the nose, in that order against the floor, lift your head and toss head back. Remember, the *bhujanga* or the cobra does not have any hands, and yet manages to raise its hood and we need to imitate that. But many texts show the use of palms!
- Take minimal help from our palms, unlike in the previous asana, and lift your head and shoulders and toss head back
- Cross your fingers on your back and place the crossed fingers on your hips.
- Stretch your hands in that position and pin down your hips with the crossed fingers and palms.
- Ensure that your body below the waist is fully stretched out and your toes are pointed and together.
- Stay in this posture for 30 seconds or longer, if you can, and lower the upper torso down, landing the head on the chin, scraping the nose on the floor and resting the head on the forehead, as in *Sva:na:sana*. Try to breathe normally throughout.

Chapter 15

Yoga and Pregnancy

Child birth education and prenatal yoga are spreading across India and America. Pregnancy brings about physiological, psychological and hormonal changes in women. They also undergo much stress related to these changes as well as due to the social and work environment. Normal stress gets intensified and so may have a more adverse effect in pregnancy than in normal state, both on the fetus as well as on the mother to be. None can forget that the mother's DNA registers all that she experiences and the same DNA gets inherited by the baby. More clinical evidence is coming up discretely in view of the nature of pregnancy, and the appropriateness of not being experimental about reducing labor pain, of the need to increase maternal comfort, and ensure safe delivery of healthy babies. One of such discrete studies is from Thailand and dated 2007. It was, as a matter of fact a randomized controlled study by Chuntharapat et al.[154] The objectives of this study was to examine if yoga exercise during pregnancy has a beneficial impact on comfort, labor pain and birth outcomes. The sample consisted of only primigravid (first time pregnant) Thai women divided into two equal groups: experimental and control.

Six one-hour long yoga sessions were administered for the experimental group at a prescribed 2-week period of gestation or trimester. Several gadgets were used to gauge maternal comfort, labor pain and birth outcomes. The results indicated that, compared to the control group, those exposed to yoga had higher levels of maternal comfort during labor and 2 hours post-labor and had less subject-evaluated labor pain. The experimental group had two-and-a-half hours shorter first stage of labor than the control group: mean length of first stage – 520 minutes in yoga group versus 660 minutes in control group; mean total time in labor 559 minutes in yoga group versus 684 minutes in control group.[155] As clarified by the Prenatal Yoga Center, the factors that seem to facilitate realization of yoga benefits are: "First, yoga involves synchronization of breathing awareness and muscle relaxation which decrease tension and the perception of pain. Second, yoga movements, breathing, and chanting may increase circulating endorphins and serotonin, 'raising the threshold of mind-body relationship to pain'. Third, practicing yoga postures over time alters pain pathways through the parasympathetic nervous system, decreasing one's need to actively respond to unpleasant physical sensations."

However, the Thai study pointed out that in both the groups pain increased and maternal comfort decreased with progress in labor. There were no differences between the two groups in regard to pethidine usage, labor augmentation, or new born Apgar scores at 1 and 5 minutes. The 1-minute score measures how well the baby tolerated the birth process and the 5-minute tests how the baby is doing outside the womb.

The Prenatal Center advocates prenatal yoga for ten reasons:

1. Community help is needed to get along especially when pregnant
2. Prenatal yoga alleviates aches and pains
3. Need to connect with the baby inside
4. Help align the pelvis
5. Learn physical coping skills
6. Learn emotional coping skills
7. Need much edification in prenatal yoga
8. Learn about the vital breath connection
9. Find autonomy in the delivery clinic
10. Find the pelvic floor through soft diaphragmatic breathing

More and more women seem to prefer non-pharmacological solutions to maternal depression that occurs during pregnancy. This is a critical health issue considering that the mental and physical health of both the mother and the baby to be delivered is at stake. A recent study with a meta-analysis of clinical studies of yoga intervention (YI) in maternal depression during pregnancy has much to offer in terms of evidence of effectiveness of YI. The study by Ng QX et al[156] reviewed 8 clinical studies systematically and included 6 studies with a total of 405 pregnant women. The meta-analysis applied a per-protocol analysis together with a random-effects model. The pooled standardized mean difference (SMD) from the baseline depressive score was -452 (95% CI -0.816 to 0.880, P = 0.015.) This is statistically significant beneficial effect on the mood attributable to YI. Limitations of this meta-analysis are that most trials were preliminary in nature, participants recruited had only mild depression, there was no blinding and the sample sizes were relatively small.

An earlier study by Hong Gong et al (2015)[157] was also a meta-analysis to look into the effects of YI on prenatal depression. After thorough search the researchers settled on six RCTs up to July 2014. The sample size added up to 375 pregnant women in the age group of 20-40 years. Structured Clinical Interview for DSM-IV and the Center for Epidemiological Studies Depression Scale were used to diagnose depression. The results were, compared to standard prenatal care, standard antenatal exercises, social support and their like, in the yoga groups depression was reduced to a statistically significant level: SMD -0.59, 95% CI -0.94 to -0.25, p = 0.0007. In a subgroup analysis, symptoms of depression in prenatally depressed women were also lower (SMD, -0.46; CI, -0.90 to -0.03; p = 0.04) And among non-depressed women (SMD, -0.87; CI, -1.22 to -0.52; p < 0.00001) symptoms of depression were statistically significantly lower in yoga group than that in control group.

Yet another subgroup was formed on the basis of type of YI. There were two types: the physical-exercise-based yoga and integrated yoga. The latter, besides physical exercises, included pranayama, meditation or deep relaxation. The results showed that the level of depression was significantly decreased in the integrated yoga group (SMD, -0.79; CI, -1.07 to -0.51; p < 0.00001) but not significantly reduced in physical-exercise-based yoga group (SMD, -0.41; CI, -1.01 to -0.18; p = 0.17). The study upheld the validity of YI for prenatal maternal depression.

According to a more recent study, it is encouraging that 38 percent of women in the age group 28-33 years practice yoga. This 2012 study looked into evidence of YI in pregnancy from three randomized control trials (RCT) and three controlled trials.[158] The findings of this study were that yoga is well indicated for pregnant women and improves all outcomes related to pregnancy, labor and birth. The yoga practices imparted to pregnant ladies were postures (*asana*), breathing exercises (*pranayama*), concentration/meditation (*dharana/ dhyana*), deep relaxation/yoga sleep (*nidra*), lecture/ counseling, anatomy and chanting.

Several of the six studies provided holistic approach to promoting health of pregnant women that would stand in good stead on a daily basis. One of the highlights of the study was its unequivocal endorsement that yoga reduces inflammatory markers, lowers heart rate, and improves physical fitness. These benefits add up to promote behavioral changes and psychosocial functions contributing to much better reactivity to stress and pain, the two blatant factors in pregnancy. On the down side, because the studies were not being double blinded and not all randomized, the conclusions could not be generalized. The study suggested a prenatal yoga program that results in benefits during pregnancy as well as throughout labor and birth outcomes. For the sake of the health and wellbeing of future generations this counsel needs to be taken earnestly.

YI in pregnancy at all stages has proved itself to have highly salutary effects both for the wellness of the mother and wholesome health of the baby, the future citizen.

Chapter 16

Yoga and The Elderly

The main health problem with the elderly is that they, as a group embrace the wisdom of group think that aging is uniformly the same, regardless whether you are John or Jane Doe or someone that anticipates the predicaments that come with age and takes action to mitigate aging with age-old techniques including yoga and belly breathing. Group-think passes on the wisdom of the past, but does nothing to encourage initiatives and action to prolong youth or ward off the quandaries of aging. There is no divine compulsion to submit oneself to the plights of old age. It only requires preplanned strategies including diet, exercises, moderation in emotions and detachment. Be that as it may, no one denies the role of confounding factors including as yet incomplete or inexplicable or pure bizarre geriatric medical events .

Yet another imperative is that persons desirous of being different from the run of elderly should acquire a good working knowledge of anatomy and physiology of one's body. This helps recognize predictor signals from the heart, lungs, kidneys, brain, or any other part and visualize health issues and diagnose them before they become problems. At least the frequency of falling sick as we get old can be brought down as well as the severity of the illness. Also falling sick is not inescapable every time.

The number of elderly people with increasing risk of dependency needing accommodation in assisted living centers is on the rise due to demographic factors such as downward trends in fertility and mortality as well as long life expectancies. This does not mean that the quality of life of these seniors is anything to be happy about. Elderly population aged 60 years or more, in India has gone up from 7.4 percent in 2000 to about 11 percent currently, the rates differing from state to state.[159] The projections are that the elderly population in India would go up from 7.6 million in 2001 to 137 million by 2021.

In the US, there were 40.3 million aged 65 years or older in 2010 and this went up to 54 million by July 2019. Much of the increase came from Baby Boomers born between 1946-1964. According to the Census Bureau the size of the 65-and-older population grew by over a third since 2010, outdoing all other age groups in the size of the increase.[160]

As people age, secretions of Growth Hormone (GH) and dehydroepiandrosterone sulfate (DHEAS) are expected to decline. However exponents of yoga have believed that that this process associated with aging can be slowed or delayed by the regular practice of yoga which would restore the normal endocrinological functions of the human body. In order to test this claim a study[161] was undertaken with 23 persons (15 male and 8 female) in the yoga group and 22 persons in the waitlisted control group (15 male and 7 female). The mean age range was 41 – 53 years. The yoga group was imparted integrated yoga practice daily for six days a week for 12 weeks. The control group carried on with routine activities. There were measurements of standing height, body weight, BMI, and basal level GH and DHEAS before commencement and at end of six weeks and 12 weeks of yoga training. The results showed (Figure 15) that compared to baseline data, there was significant increase in GH and DHEAS for both males and females in the yoga group. This was not the case with the control group. The conclusion was yoga promotes healthy aging.

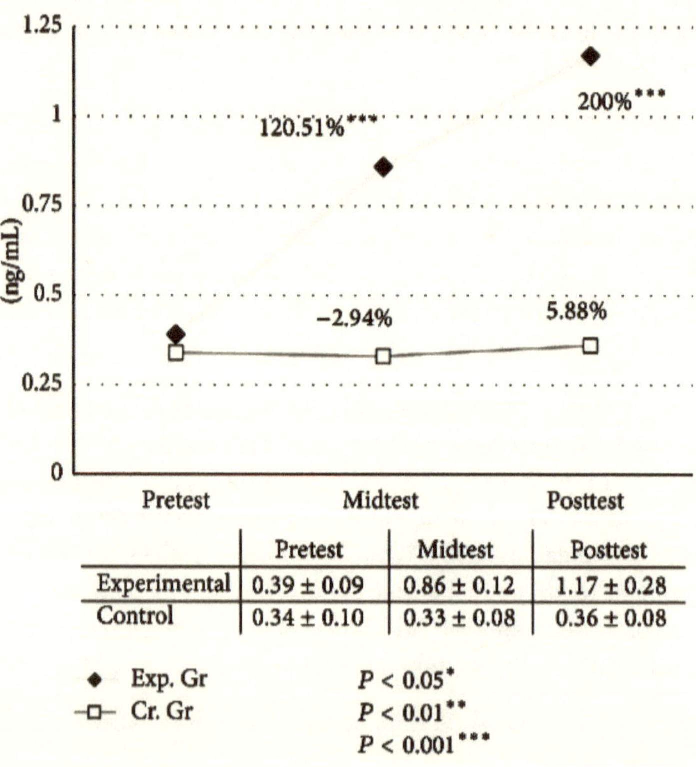

	Pretest	Midtest	Posttest
Experimental	0.39 ± 0.09	0.86 ± 0.12	1.17 ± 0.28
Control	0.34 ± 0.10	0.33 ± 0.08	0.36 ± 0.08

◆ Exp. Gr	$P < 0.05^*$
–□– Cr. Gr	$P < 0.01^{**}$
	$P < 0.001^{***}$

Fig.15: GH and DHEAS Output Among the Elderly

Source: Chatterjee et al (2014)

The increase in growth hormone and DHEAS in the yoga group as compared to the control group is impressive. This is the case whether one looks at the percentages or the actuals.

Aging and Gene Factors

Aging happens not chronologically with each birthday, but according to how much even-minded people are in both difficulties and in wholesome progress. Slow or fast aging happens also according to physical fitness and mental equanimity. As has been noted under different chapters, for instance, being overweight definitely contributes to hastening aging, as does depression, stress, worrying, loneliness, and smoking. Both in the opening chapters and on Genes, some of these factors were discussed with reference to telomeres. These stretches of DNA and proteins at the end of chromosomes shortens with aging. Second there is the genotype. Managing gene function or phenotype could contribute to aging at a slower rate.

Suppose the genotype, the epigenetic clock, of a person states an early death by heart attack at around 60 years. Be that as it may, gene expression or the gene function can be managed through yoga to adjourn the bad event. Besides telomeres and the epigenetic clock, three other predictors of aging according to a recent study are a) transcriptomes or the genetic code b) metabolomics which tells about the metabolites or small molecules produced during metabolizing and c) proteomic clock measuring the amount of proteins in blood by the metabolic processes.[162] The study found little correlation ($r < 0.2$) between the predictors and there was little overlap. It also suggested that the composite index of all five clocks brought out more distinct relations with health determinants than individual clocks. This inference is suggested by the large effect sizes of the composite index and the low correlation between aging indicators.

The onset of age heralds several physical and mental challenges people. This more or less, depends upon how well life is being led (HRQoL), how nutritious is the diet, how health-conscious the aging person is especially in terms of eschewing smoking, drinking and related addictions, how much time is spent working out the mind and the body, the nature of the bionetwork in which a person resides, and so forth. Often observers feel that much of the health care edifice is mainly for the aged considering the epidemiological dimensions of diseases such as cardiovascular sickness, diabetes, obesity, rheumatic arthritis, psychiatric disorders including dementia, cognitive impairment and so forth, besides subnormal social-economic situations like being single without support from family, not to speak of impaired vision and hearing. There is also impairment of mobility. This is a rigmarole encountered frequently whether in India or the USA. The COVID-19 infectious illness has shown that the aged are more vulnerable to it thanks to the compromised immune defense in most elderly persons, including prime ministers and presidents and others lower down the hierarchy.

Health Related QoL

In this setting of special care for the elderly there has been an interesting controlled study with block randomization to check if yoga intervention would improve quality of life (QOL) and improve the sleep quality of those living in old age homes.[163] The QOL of the subjects was evaluated with World Health Organization Quality of Life Best Available Techniques (BAT) Reference (WHOQOL-BREF). The sleep quality was with reference to the Pittsburgh Sleep Quality Index. There were recordings at two points of time: the baseline and after 6 months of yoga exercises. After randomly selecting nine elderly homes, 120 elderly persons were assigned to a yoga group (n = 62) and a waitlist group (n = 58). For the yoga group there was daily yoga practice for a month, weekly practice for 3 months and a push for yoga practice without supervision for 6 months. There was no intervention in the case of persons in the waitlist group.

Repeated measures Analysis of covariance (ANCOVA) and independent t-test were used to measure the difference in outcome measures both at baseline and after 6 months. Even after controlling for higher number of years of formal education in the yoga group, there was significant improvement in all the domains of QOL and total sleep quality of the elderly in the old age homes.

The summary results are in the Table below: RMANCOVA for QOL and total sleep quality (intent-to-treat analysis after imputation by LOCF method) between yoga and waitlist group.

Table 15: Yoga improves Basic Parameters

Variable	Group	Mean (Standard Deviation)		f	P-Value
	(*N* = 120)	Baseline	6th Month		
Physical Health QOL	Yoga	52.21 (14.55)	59.56(12.04)	55.01	<0.001
	Waitlist	57.79 (13.92)	51.41 (17.54)		
Psychological Health QOL	Yoga	55.73 (10.54)	61.27 (10.33)	35.92	<0.001

Variable	Group	Mean (Standard Deviation)		f	P-Value
	Waitlist	55.53 (9.79)	52.33 (11.21)		
Social Relationships QOL	Yoga	55.42 (15.11)	62.63 (10.67)	11.33	0.001
	Waitlist	56.41 (9.98)	57.52 (10.50)		
Environment QOL	Yoga	68.74 (12.76)	72.00 (10.74)	4.39	0.038
	Waitlist	59.76 (9.36)	60.24 (9.52)		
Total Sleep QOL	Yoga	7.65 (3.36)	6.87 (3.10)	12.25	0.001
	Waitlist	8.19 (3.46)	8.78 (3.77)		
(df =1, 117); RMANCOVA – Repeated measures analysis of covariance; QOL – Quality of Life; LOCF – Last observation carried forward					

Source: Hariprasad VR et al Effects of yoga intervention on sleep and quality-of- life in elderly: A randomized controlled trial." Indian journal of psychiatry vol. 55,Suppl 3 (2013): S364-8. doi:10.4103/0019-5545.116310

Research efforts need to be continued to be made as part of pathogenesis to unravel geriatric inexplicables like arthritis, Alzheimer's, vulnerabilities to virus such as the Corona virus, cancers, diabetes, cardiac disease, genetic clocks, osteoporosis, and so forth. It is also necessary for each person to discover his/her very own golden mean between retirement and active life, avoiding excesses and deficiencies, need for avoiding pointlessness in old age, and more positively having a great purpose. Coursing through these factors there could be a path to healthy longevity. If happier people live longer than less happy people, should we not opt for being happier? See the Epilogue that follows.

Epilogue: Cheerfulness and Wellness

Santosha or Cheerfulness - Key Ingredient for Health

The second *Niyama* or tenet of yoga is *Santosha* or Cheerfulness. There is ample clinical and other evidence to show hilarity and bonhomie are extremely critical for wellness and longevity. This was dealt with in Chapter 6 at some length. Persons enjoying a sense of wellness and 'positive affect' live longer. Positive affect is the characteristic of a person subjectively feeling positive moods such as alertness, enthusiasm, goodwill, happiness, and *joie de vivre*. It is related to good cheer and pleasure-seeking. Happier persons lived longer than less happy persons. This is the finding of a 2016 study entitled Happiness and Longevity in the United States.[164] The scholars of this study employed General Social Survey-National Death Index dataset and Cox proportional hazards (CPH) models to reveal that overall, happiness resonates and is associated with longer lives among U.S. adults. Compared to people who are '**very**' happy, the risk of death is higher among '**pretty**' happy people by six percent (the 95% confidence interval is 1.01 – 1.22), and 14% higher among those '**not**' happy (CI 1.06 – 1.22). CPH models, are essentially regression models, which examine the association between one or more multiple predictor variables and survival time of patients.

These results are net of marital status, socioeconomic status, census division, and religious attendance. In other words, the results are adjusted for these factors which could be confounders. The study also concluded that after their far-reaching findings, social science and health researchers can hereafter use happiness as a stand-alone indicator of well-being. Having a sense of purpose in life also adds to longevity. This is truer among older people.

It makes sense therefore to make all public policies in favor of promoting happiness though there could be initial problems in defining the word happiness. At times it may be a moot point if such a health policy would heal a person from sickness because by prioritizing happiness, it may be compromising on say a bitter medicine or surgery that may be healing, but not increasing happiness.

There is no doubt, the time dimension specified as well as how broad a connotation happiness is given, would induce one's concurrence in this regard.

Happiness does seem to protect individuals from falling sick, and thus increase longevity. Good health also makes people happy and improves chances of living longer. The causality between factors like happiness and long life could be established by noting that happy persons' immune systems stay strong and prevent sickness. There is exciting new evidence in this regard.[165]

Human Body a Hologram of the Universe

A happy disposition appears to be favored by the bio-ecosystem as a homeostatic natural state. Human predicament seems to want all to be happy. There are sound reasons for it! The human body is, after all, a hologram of the universe, composed of all 118 elements contained in the Periodic Table of Chemical Elements such as carbon, hydrogen, oxygen, iron, copper, and scores of others from actinium to zirconium. Whether these chemicals are found in abundance or small traces in the body, we are inextricably a product of nature and governed to a significant extent by the laws of biochemistry. The laws are uninfringeable if we desire to thrive as humans. Thus oxygen, one of the elements, is indispensable for human survival, as is hydrogen which combines with oxygen to give us water, another crucial item without which there can be no life. One can say more or less the same for the other elements, an integral part of humans. Nature seems to have grand ambitions for humans, just as for the Redwood Tree or the tiger. The implications are that the human body has the potential of extraordinary achievements and performance, particularly in a *satvika* culture and setting. Unfortunately it can become diminished like in a *rajasa* or worse still, *tamasa* setting. The default nature of humans could possibly be *satvika*, to enable them make civilizational advances. This does not deny the *raison d'etre* of rajasa and tamasa characteristics say in a sumo wrestler!.

Santosha is one of the five *Niyamas* prescribed in yoga, along with *Shoucha, Swadhyaya, Tapas and Iswara Pranidhana. (Meanings of these terms are given elsewhere.)* And yet, everywhere there is much distress and unhappiness. Some people seem to have forgotten to smile, or their life has been so miserable that they didn't have the time and wherewithal to smile. Grief can be very infectious especially when we are all part of the one large human family! *(Vasudeiva kutumbakam!)* But the good news is that joy too can be equally contagious, as a matter of fact, more than sadness. There is great wisdom in being part of the laughing club. The poet Ella Wilcox wrote: "Laugh, and the world laughs with you; weep, and you weep alone." Chapter 6 dealt with Laughter as Medicine (page 62)

Yogic Wisdom

When we are angry, bitter, emotionally upset, negative in any way, even vengeful, we are basically forgetting one of the fundamental characteristics of a wise human being: being detached from outcomes, even while being neck deep in worldly (*loukika*) transactions. However, there is a scientific (health) reason why we need to maintain equanimity of the mind, regardless of the provocation, the magnitude of the failure, loss, or sorrow. As a matter of fact, scientifically and physiologically speaking, it may be better to err on the side of celebration, exhilaration and happiness (in moderation) rather than on the side of grief, sadness, or what is worse, depression.

When the word *Sukha* was coined or minted, it actually defined the meaning of the word. In Sanskrit language prefix *Su* means good and *kha* means freedom or space. Together, the total meaning is good space. Here good space refers to the space within and without. We all want free space or total mental and physical freedom, and resist piling on each other like in the adage: 'packed like sardines'! There is no space when we stand in line for anything. Time slips away. We just watch helpless. We would be more comfortable if we could all have ample mental and physical elbow and leg room wherever we go and the time to boondoggle or indulge in what is of utmost interest. Similarly, *duh* in *duhkha* means inadequate, and *kha* again has the same meaning.

Sukha and Duhkha

Sukha is the 'comfort zone' we speak of, with a psychosomatic variation to it. There is also a yogic, inner physical meaning for *sukha*: the comfortable space within our own body, between body parts, and particularly in the rib cage that houses our cardio-vascular (heart + lungs) system. Inside the rib cage the heart is wedged between the right and left lungs. There is just enough space for the lungs to inflate like a balloon when we take a deep breath. When there is *duhkha* or grief, gloom or sadness, the skeletal-muscular structure of the upper part of the body, including the rib cage, tightens and even shrinks, reducing the space for the lungs. When we are cheerless we shrink the lung's *sukha!* People experiencing grief are unable to take a deep breath. When this occurs, there is not enough oxygen flowing to the trillions of cells in the body that must be nourished to stay healthy. The cells quickly begin to weaken without adequate oxygen. People who grieve thus have a double whammy of loss, not just whatever sad event they have suffered which made them sad in the first place, but also the weakening of their body!

A certain amount of grief in the wake of loss is natural but if a person stays sad for a long time the body begins to suffer under the "weight" of this continued constriction. The respiratory (breathing in and out) system loses its vitality or zing. That in turn adversely affects the digestive system, the circulatory (blood) system, the nervous system, the reproductive system, and of course our mental abilities. The functional integrity of our body and mind is then in jeopardy.

Endocrine System Makes us a Biochemical Factory

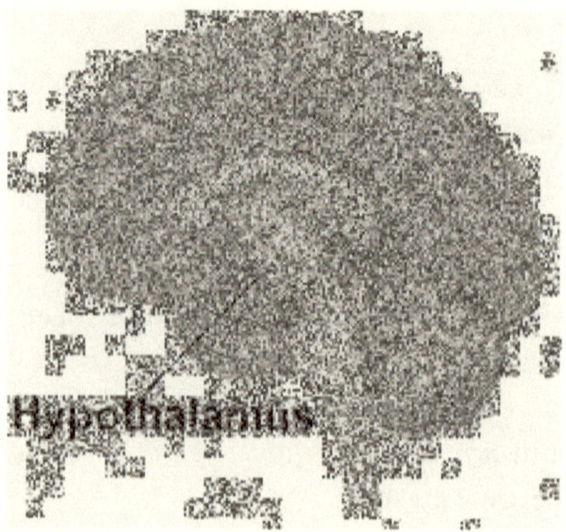

Fig 16: Hypothalamus, the Antenna Inside the Brain

Source:www.daviddarling.info

When we are physically or mentally suffering on account of grief, there is another equally critical development happening inside us. The endocrine gland called the hypothalamus, the size of a grape just above the brain stem, serves both as an antenna catching all external waves by way of sensory perception, but also as a bridge between the nervous system and the biochemical body which consists of the hormone and enzyme producing endocrine glands. The hypothalamus conveys negative happenings and feelings to the master endocrine gland, the pituitary gland. This small gland is located just below the hypothalamus at the base our brain. Any sad or negative news affects the pituitary. It does not feel up to its critical functions, and does not seem to do as good a job of monitoring everything going on in the body. In particular it becomes sloppy in hormone production and its management. It gets lax also in giving instructions to its secondary endocrine glands, the thyroid, parathyroid, the thymus, the adrenal glands, the liver, the pancreas and others regarding the release of precise quantities of the 20 or more bio-chemicals (hormones with names like Cortisol, TRH, CRH, GH, TSH, Testosterone, Dopamine, Oxytocin, Endorphin, Insulin, Somatostatin, Serotonin, Melatonin and so forth) into the blood stream. This means that the bio-chemical factory that keeps us alive and functioning at our best, slackens. For example, the pancreatic cells become sluggish due to the pituitary gland's listlessness. Pancreas slow down and there is not enough insulin produced to help digest sugar in our food. If blood sugar levels stay high, over time, diabetes may set in. Thus grief does not just make eyes teary but if prolonged it may even ruin our sound health.

One of the secrets of happiness is to learn to tap the parasympathetic nervous system through deep breathing, rather than augur the fight or flight condition spiking up the adrenal levels in the body. This calls for a better appreciation of the yogic message that breath is the bridge between the body and the mind which helps reduce the H-P-A activation and the generation of cortisol, and reduce the dominance of the stress-induced sympathetic nervous system or the limbic brain.

Joy, on the other hand, can trigger a beneficial chain reaction in our body just as sadness triggers a detrimental domino result. When experiencing joy the bio-chemical factory starts working at peak efficiency and the body parts are firing on all cylinders! The body is in great shape and you are in the pink of health! So watch out for intelligences that are generally negative and are depressing. Instead strive to spread good and true news fast, something that makes everyone smile ear to ear! Focus on news that is uplifting so that it brings happiness and spreads joy. With Nature herself as our life cohort, dark clouds should not be a problem! Vigorous yogic health will help us handle all events effortlessly, even when we perceive them as negative!

The Lotus (*punkaja* in Sanskrit) symbolism in yoga is rich. It is the driving force behind yoga pressuring us to stay happy and infect others with good cheer. The *punkaja* has its stems in muddy quagmire. (*punka in Sanskrit is* quagmire, *ja* is born. Born in quagmire), but by turning to sun, the source of all light, it blossoms out delightfully, in sharp contrast with its origin. Human life on earth could be as muddy and swampy as that of the lotus, but even that life can be as noble and worthwhile to society by turning to knowledge of one's own self.

Annexure - A Yoga Primer

What is Yoga?

Yoga is for all people, without exception, regardless of age. However, for the immense health benefits it brings, there is a compelling need to impart the knowledge of yoga to children ages 5 to 16 years. Yoga instruction can be imparted even earlier, if they can stay on the instruction and do the exercises. Of course, seeing the adults around them doing yoga is the most powerful way to introduce children to the practices and wisdom of yoga. As the old saying goes: like father, like son. It has a demonstration effect. The sooner they learn, the better it is for them because they learn about the anatomy and physiology of their mind and body and develop healthy habits. They are successful in school and in the community. It could be the best incentive to stay on yoga. They grow up with the knowledge of what an awesome bio-chemical factory the body is; how amazingly in concert the mind and the body function with the Spirit, and how to support and maintain the body and mind so that they are squeaky clean and vigorous, with all things working out fine! In view this, **the very *first* lesson in any yoga curriculum should be this holistic way of looking at ourselves, discovering that the mind, body and the spirit are working together** impeccably like a harmonious trillion-piece orchestra making perfectly glorious music! Trillion? Yes, there are more than 6-7 trillion cells in the human body; they connect with trillions of other cells. They orchestrate with sparkling brilliance! Just in order to lift a finger, the coordination of some 14 million cells and neurons is needed. How much more of them need to connect for solving problems in quantum mechanics or the seven Millennium Prize problems in mathematics?

When children and others acquire and own this yoga-based knowledge, they are empowered like never before. As they age, their yoga practice will become even more helpful in preventing them from falling sick. And should they become sick, they will be in the know of what simple exercises they can do to get well sooner than later. A young person who practices yoga regularly will be able to develop a strong immune system that is well equipped to vigorously repel viral, bacterial and fungal attacks on the body. Also, during sickness the yoga practice promotes the body's self-correcting ability through a process known as homeostasis, with or without medication and other interventions. Children will be able to rely on this wisdom and learn for themselves how simple it is to remain in rugged mental and physical health. This is the reason sage *Apasthamba Rishi* prescribed that *brahmmopadesham* (initiation into Vedic scriptures along with the orthodox thread ceremony for boys) should be imparted ideally by the age of 7 or 8 years of age. The teachings should include the elements of *pranayama,* or breathing exercises, and *asanas.* The breathing and asana exercises become integral part of the *sandhya* or the 3-times a day prayer.

It is advisable not to teach any brand name forms of yoga at the beginner level. The lessons should be generic, (plain vanilla!) yoga as they have come down to us for several millennia. There are of course many individual outstanding teachers with their own distinct styles and *ghara:nas.* The author of this article finds that it is sagacious to combine the best features of all great teachers and offer a best practices yoga that is steeped in tradition. We teach this traditional way at our Temple yoga class which has been offering yoga instruction without a break for the past 29 years, since 1992 to be exact.

Synergy

In simple terms, Yoga is yoking the mind, body and spirit in such a way that the practitioner can experience synergy with the combined effect being greater than the sum of the parts. With apologies to Pythagoras, and thanks to yoga, it is $a^2 + b^2 > C^2$ and not $a^2 + b^2 = C^2$!

It is imperative that the first lesson in a beginner's core yoga class should be one of acquainting him or her **with *Ashtanga (eight limbs) Yoga.*** Each one of the eight is important, depending upon your progress along the yoga learning curve. Yama and Niyama are the starting point for the beginner and Dhyana and Samadhi for those at the XYZ stage of Yoga, already experts in the first six limbs including Pratyahara and Dharana.

1. *Yama (Five* necessary philosophical underpinnings such as *nonviolence, truthfulness, non-covetousness or not yearning for anything, moderation, and non-grabbing of others' credits or property)*
2. *Niyama* (Five Rules of Yoga discipline such as *body-mind cleanliness, cheerfulness, focused learning all through life, reflection and meditation, and theism)*
3. *A:sana – Sthoola and Sukshma:* Heavy-duty and Subtle body exercises

4.   ***Pranayama:*** Breathing exercises
5.   ***Pratyahara:*** Withdrawal of five senses from non-essentials such as irrelevant entertainment, chatter or gossip.
6.   ***Dharana:*** mental focus on specifics
7.   ***Dhyana:*** meditation riveted on priority items and activity
8.   ***Samadhi:*** total immersion in desired activity or integration with the Universal Intelligence or Consciousness (Chinmaya)

The last three limbs 6, 7 and 8 are intuitive; and a yoga practitioner will learn them instinctively after mastering the first five. Each one of the first five is a prerequisite for the next limb. For instance, *Yama* and *Niyama* are prerequisites for sound learning and practice of *A:sana*. *Yamas* are the moral imperatives such as *Satyam vada* (Speak the truth), *dharmam chara* (Be Righteous), and they number five (abbreviation ASABA): *Ahimsa, Satya, Astheya, Brahmacharya, and Aparigraha* (meanings given above). These are the rules of conduct for dealing with the world and its people. Turning inwards, to deal with our inner self or oneself, there are another five *Niyamas* or rules: *Santosha (happiness and cheerfulness as a default mental state, the Epilogue Chapter in this book), Soucha or cleanliness in and out, Svadhya:ya or learning for life, Ta:pa or discarding irrelevancies,* and *Iswara Pranidhana or faith in God.* (See meanings above.) Imbibing the *Yamas* and *Niyamas* is perhaps the most difficult part of Yoga. The rest, relatively speaking, are much easier. But Asana and Pranayama help accomplish Yamas and Niyamas. Whoever masters these, regardless of the current situation, will always be cheerful, with a pure smile on the face, and with a supremely happy "been there, done that" relaxed feel! This radiant smile is very infectious! Such a Yoga person makes the world a better place for all.

In the area of *Asana*, it is good to keep in mind that there are hundreds of *asanas* and numerous variations of most of them. One can spend an entire life-time learning them, but that is not necessary. There are composite asanas such as Chakrasana, Dhanurasana, Halasana, Sarvangasana, Surya Namaskar (sun salutation), each one of which brings to the practioner the benefits several individual asanas, somewhat reducing the need for doing constituent asanas of the composites. Of course, each asana has a well-defined rationale, especially in Chikitsa.

What are missing in this Yoga Syllabus are a) Mudras b) Yoga kriyas such as Jyoti trataka, Dhouti, Neti, and so forth c) Yoga Diet for fostering more Satvaguna rather than Rajoguna or Thamoguna and d) Meditation. Yoga way of life leads to a rational holistic life guaranteeing happiness. You are at peace with yourself, the world and its people, enjoying much leverage to change them for the better.

Yoga Basics

Beginners' Yoga can consist of exercises that are both easy and somewhat difficult, rather than just easy exercises. Remember chair exercises, and sukshma (subtle) exercises practiced by less flexible adults? They too have a place for a segment of the population. Once children acquire proficiency in asanas their bodies will remember them because yoga memories get embedded in the mind. Even after a lapse of decades after practicing the yoga exercises, and perhaps forgetting the very names of those exercises, they will still be able to pick them back up and do them, after good rehearsals of course!

Each person is different from the other, and so is the body structure, bio-chemistry and needs. So personalize your practice according to your own capabilities, body-mind needs, listening all the time to your mind/body, simultaneously pushing/pressuring them to go beyond the frontiers of capability. After all it is imperative that we need to get to the next higher level of yoga, not just because of new viruses and new diseases, besides the old formidable ones, but also because we want to be nobler still!

After this theoretical introduction the teacher imparts training in a) Bhastrika (Bellows) b) Nadi shodana pranayama (alternate nostril breathing) and c) three-phase shavasana (Corpse pose). These three exercises are repeated at the end of every class and they signal closure of that yoga session. This 3-exercise dose of yoga by itself, if done right, is indeed a potent prophylactic as well as medicine for numerous physical and mental health issues, and otherwise, an elixir for long happy life along the non H-P-A route which is the PSN system. There is no hyperbole here!

Temple Yoga Core Curriculum

The *second* imperative lesson in a beginner's core yoga class should be one of acquainting him or her with *Ashtanga Yoga* or the eight limbs detailed above.

In view of the fact that there are several excellent books on yoga asanas it has been decided to not come up with a section on yoga asanas. Also those interested may refer to AYUSH Ministry's the Common Yoga Protocol used on the occasion of the International Day of Yoga. The web address is given at Endnote 1.

Endnotes and References

1. AYUSH, Government of India, Common Yoga Protocol accessed at https://yoga.ayush.gov.in/yoga/common-yoga-protocol, International Day of Yoga 2019 | Common Yoga Protocol (CYP) | ENGLISH | FULL HD

2. Maria Cohut (2020), Yoga Keeps the Mind and Body Young, 22 clinical trials show, *Medical News Today,* available at https://www.medicalnewstoday.com/articles/325374#Yoga-has-great-potential-to-improve-health

3. Cartwright T. et al. Yoga Practice in the UK: A cross-sectional survey of motivations, health behaviors and benefits. Accessed from - https://bmjopen.bmj.com/content/bmjopen/10/1/e031848.full.pdfv

4. Hagins M, et al, Research Perspective Bridging Yoga Therapy and Scientific Research, INTERNATIONAL JOURNAL OF YOGA THERAPY – No. 22 (2012) 5

5. Bussing A. et al. Effects of Yoga on Mental and Physical Health, A Short Summary of Reviews, accessed at https://www.hindawi.com/journals/ecam/2012/165410/

6. Woodyard C. Exploring the therapeutic effects of yoga and its ability to increase quality of life. *Int J Yoga*. 2011;4(2):49-54. doi:10.4103/0973-6131.85485

7. Mohammad A, et al, Biological markers for the effects of yoga as a complementary and alternative medicine. J Complement Integr Med. 2019 Feb 7;16(1):/j/jcim.2019.16.issue-1/jcim-2018-0094/jcim-2018-0094.xml. doi: 10.1515/jcim-2018-0094. PMID: 30735481.

8. Yoga Statistics: Surprising Data on the Growth of Yoga accessed at https://www.eventbrite.com/blog/yoga-statistics-demographics-market-growth-trends-ds00/

9. Stephens I. Medical Yoga Therapy, https://www.medicalnewstoday.com/articles/325374#Yoga-has-great-potential-to-improve-health Woodyard C. Exploring the therapeutic effects of yoga and its ability to increase quality of life. *Int J Yoga*. 2011;4(2):49-54. doi:10.4103/0973-6y, Children (Basel). 2017. Published online 2017 Feb 10. doi: 10.3390/children4020012 Feb; 4(2): 12.

10. Ornish D, et al, Effect of comprehensive lifestyle changes on telomerase activity and telomere length in men with biopsy-proven low-risk prostate cancer: 5-year follow-up of a descriptive pilot study. Lancet Oncol. 2013 Oct;14(11):1112-1120. doi: 10.1016/S1470-2045(13)70366-8. Epub 2013 Sep 17. PMID: 24051140.

11. Rathore, Mrithunjay, and et al, "Implication of Asana, Pranayama and Meditation on Telomere Stability." *International journal of yoga* vol. 11,3 (2018): 186-193. doi:10.4103/ijoy.IJOY_51_17

12. Kumar SB, et al, Telomerase activity and cellular aging might be positively modified by a yoga-based lifestyle intervention. *J Altern Complement Med*. 2015; 21:370–2.

13. Vazza F., et al, The Strange Similarity of Neuron and Galaxy Networks, accessed at https://nautil.us/issue/50/emergence/the-strange-similarity-of-neuron-and-galaxy-networks

14. Vaidya A. interview with Padmanabhan C. The Mind, a Cow, and the Challenges of Cancer. Wire magazine. Accessed at https://thewire.in/culture/mind-cows-challenges-of-cancer

15. Vaidya. A. Coping with Corona Virus: Lessons from a Cancer Survivor, Conde Nast Traveler May 08, 2020, accessed at https://www.cntraveller.in/story/coping-with-coronavirus-lessons-cancer-survivor-kerala/

16. Pilkington K.et al.Yoga for Depression: the research evidence. Journal of Affective Disorders, 89 (1-3). pp. 13-24, December 2005, available on line at http://www.sciencedirect.com/science/journal/01650327

17. Healio News May 02, 2014,Cardiology, Perspective from Helene Glassber, Yoga may improve CVD Risk Factors, accessed from https://www.healio.com/news/cardiology/20140502/yoga-may-improve-cvd-risk-factors?utm_source=TrendMD&utm_medium=cpc&utm_campaign=Healio__TrendMD_1

18. Helliwell, JF., et al, eds. 2020. World Happiness Report 2020. New York: Sustainable Development Solutions Network accessible from https://worldhappiness.report/ed/2020/#read

19. Madison A. (2001) The World Economy: A Millennial Perspective, OECD, Paris 2001 ISBN 92-64-18998-X, pp.320-345

20. Stephens I. *Ibid*

21. Clarke TC, et al, Use of yoga, meditation, and chiropractors among U.S. adults aged 18 and older. NCHS Data Brief, no 325. Hyattsville, MD: National Center for Health Statistics. 2018.

22. Norberg U. Restorative Yoga, Reduce Stress, Gain energy and Find Balance, Skyhorse Publishing, Pp.4-6, Amazon Kindle Book accessed at https://www.amazon.in/Restorative-Yoga-Reduce-Stress-Balance/dp/1510705309

23. Cramer H, et al, Adverse events associated with yoga: a systematic review of published case reports and case series. PLoS One. 2013 Oct 16;8(10):e75515. doi: 10.1371/journal.pone.0075515. PMID: 24146758; PMCID: PMC3797727.

24. https://www.nccih.nih.gov/health/yoga-what-you-need-to-know

25. Mullaney T CNBC, Modern Medicine, The most common knee surgery for seniors is costly, and usually a waste, April 06, 2018, accessed at: https://www.cnbc.com/2018/04/05/knee-surgery-for-seniors-is-costly-and-usually-a-waste.html

26. Shimoga Cancer Treatment, Shri Narayana Murthy accessed at https://zenonco.io/articles-and-blogs/shimoga-cancer/#:~:text=The%20city%20is%20also%20known,known%20as%20Shimoga%20cancer%20treatment.

27. National Cancer Institute: A Story of Discovery: Natural Compound Helps Treat Breast and Ovarian Cancers. Accessed at https://www.cancer.gov/research/progress/discovery/taxol

28. Harvard Health Publishing, Corona Virus Resource Center, accessed at https://www.health.harvard.edu/diseases-and-conditions/coronavirus-resource-center

29. Nagarathna R, et al. "A Perspective on Yoga as a Preventive strategy for Coronavirus Disease 2019." *International journal of yoga* vol. 13, 2 (2020): 89-98. doi:10.4103/ijoy.IJOY_22_20

30. Nagarathna R. Ibid and PEFR Rates https://svyasa.edu.in.

31. Peng Xie, et al, Severe COVID-19: A Review of Recent Progress with a Look Toward the Future. Frontiers in Public Health, 2020; 8 DOI: 10.3389/fpubh.2020.00189

32. National Clinical Management Protocol based on Ayurveda and Yoga for the management of Covid-19" released jointly by Health and AYUSH Ministers accessed at https://pib.gov.in/PressReleseDetail.aspx?PRID=1662012

33. Mishra AS, et al (2020) Knowledge, Attitude and Practice of Yoga in Rural and Urban India, KAPY2017, A National Cluster Sample Survey, Medicines (Basel). 2020 Feb; 7(2): 8.Published online 2020 Feb 5. doi: 10.3390/medicines7020008, Accessed from https://www.ncbi.nlm.nih.gov/pmc/articles/PMC7168227/

34. Berwick MB Elusive Waste The Fermi Paradox in the US Health Care, JAMA. 2019;322(15):1458-1459. doi:10.1001/jama.2019.14610

35. Maddox KEJ et al, Editorial: Toward Evidence-Based Policy Making to Reduce Wasteful Health Care Spending, *JAMA. 2019;322(15):1460-1462. doi:10.1001/jama.2019.13977*

36. Char S. Cancer Therapies: Quantum-level Contribution of Ayurveda and Yoga Highlighted Significant Health Tech Data Exchange in Harvard meet, Medical & Clinical Research, 2018 Vol 3, Issue 7, 1-9 accessed at https://medclinres.org/pdfs/2018/cancer-therapies-quantum-level-contribution-of-ayurveda-and-yoga-highlighted-significant-health-tech-data-exchange-in-harvard-meet-mcr-18.pdf

37. Nagarathna R et al, Integrated Approach to Yoga Therapy for Positive Health, Swami Vivekananda Yoga Prakashana, Bangalore 560019, Pages 30-35 quoting from Laghu Yoga Vasishtha.

38. H. Nagendra, et al, "Cognitive Behavior Evaluation Based on Physiological Parameters among Young Healthy Subjects with Yoga as Intervention", Computational and Mathematical Methods in Medicine, vol. 2015, Article ID 821061, 13 pages, 2015. https://doi.org/10.1155/2015/821061

39. Aurora JP et al Yoga as an Intervention for the Reduction of Symptoms of Anxiety and Depression in Children and Adolescents: A Systematic Review, *Front Pediatr* 2020 Mar 13;8:78. doi: 10.3389/fped.2020.00078. eCollection 2020. Accessed from https://pubmed.ncbi.nlm.nih.gov/32232017/

40. Collins, L. Head First, The New Yorker, Sept. 21, 2009, http://www.newyorker.com/magazine/2009/09/21/head-first

41. Nall R., et al, What is the difference between Migraines and Headaches? *Healthline* August 2020, accessed from https://www.healthline.com/health/migraine/migraine-vs-headache

42. Doherty C, et al, The Difference Between Migraines and Sinus Headaches, verywell health, accessed from https://www.verywellhealth.com/sinus-infection-or-migraine-1719600

43. American Headache Society, What are Behavioral Migraine Treatment Options? Accessed at https://americanheadachesociety.org/wp-content/uploads/2019/03/Behavioral-Infographic_V3-11x14.pdf

44. WebMD, When Stress Is a Chronic Migraine Trigger, accessed at https://www.webmd.com/migraines-headaches/prevent-migraine-20/stress-triggers-chronic-migraine?ecd=wnl_gdh_112120&ctr=wnl-gdh-112120_nsl-ftn_2&mb=WPi%40zcnwSaubZhNwaNjn2%40HnVev1imbCvjLb0DevlXo%3d

45. Iyengar, BKS Yoga: The Path to Holistic Health, Dorling Kindersley Ltd., 2001. 333-4

46. John PJ, et al, Effectiveness of yoga therapy in the treatment of migraine without aura: a randomized controlled trial. Headache. 2007 May;47(5):654-61

47. Kisan, R et al. "Effect of Yoga on migraine: A comprehensive study using clinical profile and cardiac autonomic functions." *International journal of yoga* vol. 7,2 (2014): 126-32. doi:10.4103/0973-6131.133891

48. Tortora GJ et al, Principles of Anatomy and Physiology, Figure 14-2, 387

49. Vallath N. "Perspectives on yoga inputs in the management of chronic pain." *Indian journal of palliative care* vol. 16,1 (2010): 1-7. doi:10.4103/0973-1075.63127

50. Balaji PA, et al, (2012) Physiological effects of yogic practices and transcendental meditation in health and disease. N Am J Med Sci. 2012 Oct; 4(10):442-8. Accessed from https://www.ncbi.nlm.nih.gov/pmc/articles/PMC3482773/

51. Shamdasani S. (1999) Neuroscience & Psychology The Psychology of Kundalini Yoga: *Notes of the Seminar Given in 1932,* Princeton University Press accessed at https://press.princeton.edu/books/paperback/9780691006765/the-psychology-of-kundalini-yoga

52. Aiello K. A Transverse Cut: A look at C.G. Jung's English Seminar on the Kundalini Yoga, accessed at http://www.createsilence.com/bits/posts/jung.html#fn1

53. Swami Satyananda Sarawati (2013) Asana Pranayama Mudra Bandha, Yoga Publications Trust, Munger, Bihar, India, Pp.526-536

54. Pilkington K.et al.Yoga for Depression: the research evidence. Journal of Affective Disorders, 89 (1-3). pp. 13-24, December 2005, available on line at http://www.sciencedirect.com/science/journal/01650327

55. Lawrence M, Et al Yoga for stroke rehabilitation. Cochrane Database Syst Rev. 2017 Dec 8;12(12):CD011483. doi: 10.1002/14651858.CD011483.pub2. PMID: 29220541; PMCID: PMC6486003.

56. Rai D, et al. Country- and individual-level socioeconomic determinants of depression: multilevel cross-national comparison. Br J Psychiatry. 2013;202:195–203. [PubMed] [Google Scholar]

57. Dick A. et al Examining Mechanisms of Change in a Yoga Intervention for Women: The Influence of Mindfulness, Psychological Flexibility, and Emotion Regulation on PTSD Symptoms, Journal of Clinical Psychiatry, https://doi.org/10.1002/jclp.22104

58. Cramer H, et al, Yoga for anxiety: A systematic review and meta-analysis of randomized controlled trials. Depress Anxiety. 2018 Sep;35(9):830-843. doi: 10.1002/da.22762. Epub 2018 Apr 26. PMID: 29697885.

59. Kumar S, Effect of adjunct yoga therapy in depressive disorders: Findings from a randomized controlled study. Indian J Psychiatry 2019;61:592-7

60. Naveen GH, et al. Development and feasibility of yoga therapy module for out-patients with depression Indian J Psychiatry 2013;55:350-6. Accessed at http://www.indianjpsychiatry.org. Also at https://pubmed.ncbi.nlm.nih.gov/24049198/

61. Fishbein, D., et al, Behavioral and Psychophysiological Effects of a Yoga Intervention on High-Risk Adolescents: A Randomized Control Trial. *J Child Fam Stud* 25, 518–529 (2016). https://doi.org/10.1007/s10826-015-0231-6

62. National Library of Medicine – gamma Aminobutyric Acid, accessed at https://pubchem.ncbi.nlm.nih.gov/compound/gamma-Aminobutyric-acid#:~:text=Gamma-aminobutyric%20acid%20is%20a%20gamma-amino%20acid%20that%20is,monocarboxylic%20acid.%20It%20derives%20from%-20a%20butyric%20acid.

63. Streeter CC et al Thalamic Gamma Aminobutyric Acid Level Changes in Major Depressive Disorder After a 12-Week Iyengar Yoga and Coherent Breathing Intervention, PMID: 31934793, PMCID: PMC7074898 (available on 2021-03-01), DOI: 10.1089/acm.2019.0234, Accessed from https://pubmed.ncbi.nlm.nih.gov/31934793/

64. Nyer M et al A randomized controlled dosing study of Iyengar yoga and coherent breathing for the treatment of major depressive disorder: Impact on suicidal ideation and safety findings, Complement Ther Med. 2018 Apr;37:136-142. doi: 10.1016/j.ctim.2018.02.006. Epub 2018 Feb 23. et al PMID: 29609926 DOI: 10.1016/j.ctim.2018.02.006. Accessed from https://pubmed.ncbi.nlm.nih.gov/31934793/

65. Streeter CC et al Effects of yoga versus walking on mood, anxiety, and brain GABA levels: a randomized controlled MRS study, J Altern Complement Med.,. 2010 Nov; 16(11):1145-52. doi: 10.1089/acm.2010.0007. Epub 2010 Aug 19. Accessed from https://pubmed.ncbi.nlm.nih.gov/20722471/

66. For more information on the lymphatic system see: https://www.betterhealth.vic.gov.au/health/conditionsandtreatments/immune-system#:~:text=The%20immune%20system%20is%20a,it%20enters%20the%20body%20again.

67. Gopal A. et al (2011) Effect of integrated yoga practices on immune responses in examination stress – A preliminary study, International Journal of Yoga, Int J Yoga. 2011 Jan-Jun; 4(1): 26–32.doi: 10.4103/0973-6131.78178, accessed at https://www.ncbi.nlm.nih.gov/pmc/articles/PMC3099098/

68. Cozzolino, Mauro et al. "The Evaluation of a Mind-Body Intervention (MBT-T) for Stress Reduction in Academic Settings: A Pilot Study." *Behavioral sciences (Basel, Switzerland)* vol. 10,8 124. 30 Jul. 2020, doi:10.3390/bs10080124

69. Kenney MJ et al, (2014) Autonomic Nervous System and Immune System Interactions, Compr Physiol. 2014 Jul; 4(3): 1177–1200. doi: 10.1002/cphy.c130051. Accessed from https://www.ncbi.nlm.nih.gov/pmc/articles/PMC4374437/

70. Help Guide: https://www.helpguide.org/articles/mental-health/laughter-is-the-best-medicine.htm#:~:text=A%20good%2C%20hearty%20laugh%20relieves,improving%20your%20resistance%20to%20disease.

71. Ganesan K. et al 2018 Intermittent Fasting: The Choice for a Healthier Lifestyle, Cureus. 2018 Jul; 10(7): e2947. Published online 2018 Jul 9. doi: 10.7759/cureus.2947 Accessed from https://www.ncbi.nlm.nih.gov/pmc/articles/PMC6128599/

72. Holland K., Healthline accessed at https://www.healthline.com/health/obesity-facts

73. CDC&P, Adult Obesity Facts accessed at https://www.cdc.gov/obesity/data/adult.html

74. Bird E et al (2020) Veg Diet May Promote Healthy Aging, Medical News Today Newsletter, accessed at https://www.medicalnewstoday.com/articles/vegan-diet-

may-promote-healthy-aging?utm_source=newsletter&utm_medium=email&utm_campaign=MNT%20Daily%20News&utm_content=2020-07-29&utm_country=&utm_hcp=&apid=35582212

75. Pimental D, et al, (2003) Sustainability of Meat-based and Plant-based Diet and the Environment, The American Journal of Clinical Nutrition, Volume 78, Issue 3, September 2003, Pages 660S–663S, https://doi.org/10.1093/ajcn/78.3.660S

76. *Yoko Yokoyama et al JAMA Intern Med. 2014;174(4):577-587. doi:10.1001/jamainternmed.2013.14547 Accessed from* https://jamanetwork.com/journals/jamainternalmedicine/fullarticle/1832195

77. Rosenthal E (2017) An American Sickness, Penguin Press, NY. Pp. 241-261

78. Gawande A. 2009 The Cost Conundrum, The New Yorker magazine, May 25, 2009 accessed from https://www.newyorker.com/magazine/2009/06/01/the-cost-conundrum

79. Sharma H et al, Dynamic DNA Activating your Inner Energy for Better Health, Select Books, ISBN 9781590794470, available at https://lccn.loc.gov/2017040814

80. Ornish et al 2013 I*bid*

81. Sharma H 2014 cited in Sharma H and Meade JG 2018 *Ibid*

82. 82 Ornish D, et al. Effect of comprehensive lifestyle changes on telomerase activity and telomere length in men with biopsy-proven low-risk prostate cancer: 5-year follow-up of a descriptive pilot study. Lancet Oncol. 2013 Oct;14(11):1112-1120. doi: 10.1016/S1470-2045(13)70366-8. Epub 2013 Sep 17. PMID: 24051140.

83. Buric, Ivana et al. "What Is the Molecular Signature of Mind-Body Interventions? A Systematic Review of Gene Expression Changes Induced by Meditation and Related Practices." *Frontiers in immunology* vol. 8 670. 16 Jun. 2017, doi:10.3389/fimmu.2017.00670

84. Ornish D, et al, Changes in prostate gene expression in Men undergoing Intensive Nutrition and Lifestyle Intervention' Proceedings of the National Academy of Sciences, USA 2008, 105(24); 8369-8374 This case study is from Sharma et al Dynamic DNA pp. 111-112

85. Sciencing accessed at https://sciencing.com/rungs-dna-double-helix-made-of-2960.html

86. Source of much of the information on DNA here is: https://www.genome.gov/human-genome-project/Completion-FAQ#:~:text=The%20bases%20are%20adenine%20(A,nucleus%20of%20all%20our%20cells.

87. Specter M. Annals of Science, Seeds of Doubt, The New Yorker, August 25, 2014 issue.

88. Normile D Chinese scientist who produced genetically altered babies sentenced to 3 years in jail, Science Mag December 30, 2019 accessed at https://www.sciencemag.org/news/2019/12/chinese-scientist-who-produced-genetically-altered-babies-sentenced-3-years-jail

89. Reardon S. US science advisers outline path to genetically modified babies, Feb 17, 2017. Accessed from https://www.nature.com/news/us-science-advisers-outline-path-to-genetically-modified-babies-1.21474

90. Minikel E et al, Broad Institute, An Appeal for Donation for Research accessible at https://giving.broadinstitute.org/broadignite/team/eric-minikel-and-sonia-vallabh

91. Mukherjee S. The Gene, An Intimate History. Scribner, gene as a basic unit pp. 9-10, 485

92. Terry Gross interview with Siddharth Mukherjee. An Oncologist Writes 'A Biography Of Cancer' 11/17/2010 https://www.wbur.org/npr/131382460/an-oncologist-writes-a-biography-of-cancer

93. Center for Disease Control (CDC) Heart disease facts. 2016. Available at: http://www.cdc.gov/heartdisease/facts.htm

94. Manchanda SC, et al. Retardation of coronary atherosclerosis with yoga lifestyle intervention. The Journal of the Association of Physicians of India. 2000 Jul;48(7):687-694

95. Amaravathi E, et al, Yoga-Based Postoperative Cardiac Rehabilitation Program for Improving Quality of Life and Stress Levels: Fifth-Year Follow-up through a Randomized Controlled Trial. *Int J Yoga*. 2018;11(1):44-52. doi:10.4103/ijoy.IJOY_57_16

96. 92 Marshall Hagins et al 2013, Effectiveness of Yoga for Hypertension: Systematic Review and Meta-Analysis, *Evidence-Based Complementary and Alternative Medicine*, Vol. 2013, Article id 649836, https://doi.org/10.1155/2013/649836

97. Cohen DL et al Iyengar Yoga versus Enhanced Usual Care on Blood Pressure in Patients with Prehypertension to Stage I Hypertension: a Randomized Controlled Trial, Evidence-Based Complementary and Alternative Medicine Volume 2011, Article ID 546428, 8 pagesdoi:10.1093/ecam/nep130, Hindawi Publishing Corporation, accessed at https://www.academia.edu/14229510/Iyengar_Yoga_versus_Enhanced_Usual_Care_on_Blood_Pressure_in_Patients_with_Prehypertension_to_Stage_I_Hypertension_a_Randomized_Controlled_Trial?email_work_card=view-paper

98. Tyagi A. et al, Yoga and Hypertension: A Systematic Review (2013) Alternative Therapies in Health and Medicine, 2014 Accessed from https://www.ncbi.nlm.nih.gov/pubmed/24657958

99. Kumari S. et al, A Way to Control Blood Pressure: Yoga and Pranayama, International Journal of Medical Research and Pharmaceutical Sciences, Vol 3 Issue 10: October 2016 ISSN: 2394-9414, DOI 10:5281, zenodo:160692

100. Harvard Heart Letter, Yoga-based Cardiac Rehabilitation a Promising Practice? Accessed at https://www.health.harvard.edu/heart-health/yoga-based-cardiac-rehabilitation-a-promising-practice

101. Levine GN et al (2017) American Heart Association, Meditation and Cardiovascular Risk Reduction, https://www.ahajournals.org/doi/full/10.1161/JAHA.117.002218

102. Chu P et al (2014) The effectiveness of yoga in modifying risk factors for cardiovascular disease and metabolic syndrome: A systematic review and meta-analysis of randomized controlled trials, European Journal of Preventive Cardiology, 12/15/2014 Accessed from Fiin PubMed https://doi.org/10.1177/2047487314562741

103. Cramer H (2014) Healio News May 02, 2014,Cardiology, Perspective from Helene Glassber, Yoga may improve CVD Risk Factors, accessed from https://www.healio.com/news/cardiology/20140502/yoga-may-improve-cvd-risk-factors?utm_source=TrendMD&utm_medium=cpc&utm_campaign=Healio__TrendMD_1

104. Tyagi A et al, Yoga and hypertension: a systematic review, Altern Ther Health Med.,. Mar-Apr 2014;20(2):32-59. Accessed from https://pubmed.ncbi.nlm.nih.gov/24657958/

105. Bhavanani AB, et al, Comparative immediate effect of different yoga asanas on heart rate and blood pressure in healthy young volunteers. Int J Yoga 2014;7:89-95.

106. Engstrom PF et al. Physiochemical Composition of Tobacco Smoke. In: Kufe DW, et al., editors. Holland-Frei Cancer Medicine. 6th edition. Hamilton (ON): BC Decker; 2003. Available from: https://www.ncbi.nlm.nih.gov/books/NBK13173/

107. National Cancer Institute website at: https://www.cancer.gov/about-cancer/causes-prevention/risk

108. Joseph CD. Psychological supportive therapy for cancer patients. Indian J Cancer. 1983;20:268-270.

109. Bower JE et al, Yoga for Cancer Patients and Survivors, Cancer Control, July 2005, Vol.12, No. 3, Pp 165-171

110. Grady D, Dr. William Fair Dies at 66; An Expert on Prostate Cancer, New York Times, Jan 13, 2002

111. Saquib J et al Prognosis following the use of C&A medicine in women diagnosed with breast cancer, Complement Ther Med. 2012 Oct; 20(5): 283–290. https://www.ncbi.nlm.nih.gov/entrez/eutils/elink.fcgi?dbfrom=pubmed&retmode=ref&cmd=prlinks&id=22863642

112. Buffart LM et al yoga in cancer patients and survivors, a systematic review and meta-analysis of randomized controlled trials. *BMC Cancer* 12, 559 (2012). https://doi.org/10.1186/1471-2407-12-559

113. Boehm K et al. Effects of Yoga Intervention on Fatigue: A Meta-Analysis, Evidence-based Complementary and Alternative Medicine, Vol 2012, doi:10.1155/2012/124703

114. Char S. Cancer Therapies: Quantum-level Contribution of Ayurveda and Yoga Highlighted Significant Health Tech Data Exchange in Harvard meet, Medical and Clinical Research, 2018, Volume 3 | Issue 7 | 1 of 9. Accessed at https://medclinres.org/pdfs/2018/cancer-therapies-quantum-level-contribution-of-ayurveda-and-yoga-highlighted-significant-health-tech-data-exchange-in-harvard-meet-mcr-18.pdf

115. Sharma H et al. Dynamic DNA, Activating your Inner Energy for Better Health, Select Books, 2018. Table 13.1 Sound of Sama Veda and Decreased Cancer Cell Growth, Table 13.2 Hard Rock Music and Increased Cancer Cell Growth, Pp 108

116. Vapiwala N. in Char ibid. Medical and Clinical Research, 2018, Volume 3 | Issue 7 | 1 of 9

117. Raghuram, et al. "Influence of Yoga on Postoperative Outcomes and Wound Healing in Early Operable Breast Cancer Patients Undergoing Surgery." International Journal of Yoga 1.1 (2008): 33. Web.

118. Ben-Joseph AM et al. Yoga Intervention for Patients with Prostate Cancer Undergoing External Beam Radiation Therapy: A Pilot Feasibility Study, Integrative Cancer Therapies, https://doi.org/10.1177/1534735415617022, Volume: 15 issue: 3, page(s): 272-278

119. Danhauer SC, et al. Yoga for symptom management in oncology: A review of the evidence base and future directions for research. Cancer. 2019;125(12):1979-1989. doi:10.1002/cncr.31979

120. Danhauer SC, 2019 Ibid

121. Danhauer et al Outcomes of Randomized Control Trials accessed at https://www.ncbi.nlm.nih.gov/pmc/articles/PMC6541520/table/T2/)

122. Char Ibid p.4 under Bypass Monocultures

123. Agarwal V, (2007) Ayurvedic medicine for schizophrenia. Cochrane Database of Systematic Reviews CD006867.

124. Sridharan K, et al, (2011) Ayurvedic treatments for diabetes mellitus. Cochrane Database of Systematic Reviews CD008288

125. Cramer H, et al. (2017) Yoga for improving health-related quality of life, mental health and cancer-related symptoms in women diagnosed with breast cancer. Cochrane Database of Systematic Reviews CD010802

126. Rao MR et al. "Anxiolytic Effects of a Yoga Program in Early Breast Cancer Patients Undergoing Conventional Treatment: A Randomized Controlled Trial." Complementary Therapies in Medicine 17.1 (2009): 1–8. Web.

127. Subnis UB et al. "Psychosocial Therapies for Patients With Cancer: A Current Review of Interventions Using Psychoneuroimmunology-Based Outcome Measures." Integrative Cancer Therapies 13.2 (2014): 85–104. Web.

128. Vadiraja HS et al. Effects of a yoga program on cortisol rhythm and mood states in early breast cancer patients undergoing adjuvant radiotherapy: a randomized controlled trial. Integr Cancer Ther. 2009 Mar;8(1):37-46. doi: 10.1177/1534735409331456. Epub 2009 Feb 3. Erratum in: Integr Cancer Ther. 2009 Jun;8(2):195. PMID: 19190034.

129. Rao RM, et al Influence of yoga on mood states, distress, quality of life and immune outcomes in early stage breast cancer patients undergoing surgery. Int J Yoga 2008;1:11-20

130. Armer JS et al. "The Impact of Yoga on Fatigue in Cancer Survivorship: A Meta-Analysis." *JNCI cancer spectrum* vol. 4,2 pkz098. 17 Dec. 2019, doi:10.1093/jncics/pkz098

131. Taylor, T.R., *et al.* A Restorative Yoga Intervention for African-American Breast Cancer Survivors: a Pilot Study. *J. Racial and Ethnic Health Disparities* 5, 62–72 (2018). https://doi.org/10.1007/s40615-017-0342-4

132. US Geological Survey, Pharmaceuticals in Water, accessed at Pharmaceuticals in Water (usgs.gov)

133. Yuan X et al. Night Shift Work Increases the Risks of Multiple Primary Cancers in Women: A Systematic Review and Meta-analysis of 61 Articles, Cancer Epidemiol Biomarkers Prev January 1 2018 (27) (1) 25-40; DOI: 10.1158/1055-9965.EPI-17-0221. Since retracted due to methodological errors.

134. Brehm, J. W., et al, (1962). *Explorations in Cognitive Dissonance.* John Wiley & Sons Inc. https://doi.org/10.1037/11622-000, Chapter 8: Implications of Dissonance for theories of motivation.

135. Nagarathna R et al, Yoga for Bronchial Asthma, British Medical Journal, Vol. 291, October 19, 1985, Accessed from https://www.ncbi.nlm.nih.gov/pmc/articles/PMC1417003/?page=1

136. Yang ZY et al Yoga for asthma, Cochrane Database Syst Rev. 2016 Apr; 2016(4): CD010346. Published online 2016 Apr 27. doi: 10.1002/14651858. CD010346.pub2, Accessed from https://www.ncbi.nlm.nih.gov/pmc/articles/ PMC6880926/

137. Rajesh C, et al, Impact of Hatha Yoga on the Airway Resistances in Healthy Individuals and Allergic Rhinitis Patients February 2017, Indian Journal of Otolaryngology and Head & Neck Surgery 71(Suppl 86), 10.1007/s12070-017-1098-1

138. Arumugam S et al, 2016 Impact of Yoga Breathing on Total Lung Capacity of Women Soccer Players, Journal of Recent Research and Applied Studies, International Journal of Recent Research and Applied Studies, Volume 3, Issue 10 (19) October 2016

139. Malik S et al, The Physiological Responses of Yogic Breathing Techniques: A Case-Control Study, Journal of Exercise Physiology Online 14(3), June 2011, Accessed from https://www.researchgate.net/publication/235972159_The_Physiological_ Responses_of_Yogic_Breathing_Techniques_A_Case-Control_Study

140. Lawrence L. These 3 Breathing Exercises Could Turn You into a Sporting Hero, accessed at https://www.redbull.com/gb-en/breathing-techniques-for-sport#:~:text=More%20recently%2C%20in%202011%2C%20a,by%20 5%2D12%20per%20cent. 06.04.2018

141. Arumugam S. et al, 201 Ibid. https://www.researchgate.net/publication/337621352_ Impact_of_Yoga_Breathing_Exercises_on_Total_Lung_Capacity_among_ Women_Soccer_Players

142. World Health Organization Health Topics/Diabetes Accessed from https://www. who.int/health-topics/diabetes#tab=tab_1

143. Kim EI et al, Yoga for Adults with Type 2 Diabetes: A Systematic Review of Controlled Trials, J Diabetes Res. v.2016; 2016, PMC4691612 Accessed from https://www.ncbi.nlm.nih.gov/pmc/articles/PMC4691612/

144. Kim EI et al 2016 Ibid.

145. McDermott, Kelly A et al. "A yoga intervention for type 2 diabetes risk reduction: a pilot randomized controlled trial." *BMC complementary and alternative medicine* vol. 14 212. 1 Jul. 2014, doi:10.1186/1472-6882-14-212

146. Shantakumari N. et al.Effects of a yoga intervention on lipid profiles of diabetes patients with dyslipidemia, Indian Heart Journal,Volume 65, Issue 2,2013, https:// www.sciencedirect.com/science/article/pii/S0019483213000369

147. Kim EI et al. 2016 Ibid.

148. Raveendran, AV et al. "Therapeutic Role of Yoga in Type 2 Diabetes." *Endocrinology and metabolism (Seoul, Korea)* vol. 33,3 (2018): 307-317. doi:10.3803/ EnM.2018.33.3.307

149. American Chiropractic Association Back Pain Facts and Statistics, accessible at https://www.acatoday.org/Patients/What-is-Chiropractic/Back-Pain-Facts-and-Statistics#:~:text=One%2Dhalf%20of%20all%20working,back%20pain%20 symptoms%20each%20year.&text=Back%20pain%20accounts%20for%20-more,time%20worker%20in%20the%20country.&text=Experts%20estimate%20 that%20up%20to,some%20time%20in%20their%20lives.

150. Slade SC, et al, Unloaded movement facilitation exercise compared to no exercise or alternative therapy on outcomes for people with nonspecific chronic low back pain: a systematic review. 2007. In: Database of Abstracts of Reviews of Effects (DARE): Quality-assessed Reviews [Internet]. York (UK): Centre for Reviews and Dissemination (UK); 1995-. Available from: https://www.ncbi.nlm.nih.gov/books/NBK74853/

151. Chang DG et al Yoga as a treatment for chronic low back pain: A systematic review of the literature, J Orthop Rheumatol. 2016 Jan 1; 3(1): 1–8. Published online 2016 Jan 1. Accessed from https://www.ncbi.nlm.nih.gov/pmc/articles/PMC4878447/

152. 152 Lee M, et al, Effect of yoga on pain, brain-derived neurotrophic factor, and serotonin in premenopausal women with chronic low back pain. Evid Based Complement Alternat Med. 2014;2014:203173. doi: 10.1155/2014/203173. Epub 2014 Jul 10. PMID: 25120574; PMCID: PMC4120477.

153. Chang DG (2016) *Ibid*

154. Chuntharapat S, et al, Yoga during pregnancy: effects on maternal comfort, labor pain and birth outcomes. *Complement Ther Clin Pract.* 2008;14(2):105-115. doi:10.1016/j.ctcp.2007.12.007

155. Prenatal Yoga Center gives a commentary on the Thailand study. It can be accessed at: https://prenatalyogacenter.com/blog/study-yoga-during-pregnancy-effects-on-maternal-comfort-labor-pain-and-birth-outcomes/#:~:text=In%20 brief%2C%20the%20study%20provides,non%2Dyoga%E2%80%9D%20 control%20group.

156. Ng QX, et al. A meta-analysis of the effectiveness of yoga-based interventions for maternal depression during pregnancy. *Complement Ther Clin Pract.* 2019;34:8-12. doi:10.1016/j.ctcp.2018.10.016

157. Gong H, et al, Yoga for prenatal depression: a systematic review and meta-analysis. *BMC Psychiatry.* 2015;15:14. Published 2015 Feb 5. doi:10.1186/s12888-015-0393-1

158. Curtis K et al (2012) Systematic Review of Yoga for Pregnant Women: Current Status and Future Directions, Evidence-Based Complementary and Alternative Medicine, Volume 2012, Article ID 715942, 13 pages, Hindawi Publishing Corporation.

159. CSO, Ministry of Statistics, Situation Analysis of the Elderly in India 2011, accessed at http://mospi.nic.in/sites/default/files/publication_reports/elderly_in_india.pdf

160. The Census Bureau, US Government, accessed at https://www.census.gov/ newsroom/press-releases/2020/65-older-population-grows.html

161. Chatterjee S., et al, "Effect of Regular Yogic Training on Growth Hormone and Dehydroepiandrosterone Sulfate as an Endocrine Marker of Aging", Evidence-Based Complementary and Alternative Medicine, vol. 2014, Article ID 240581, 15 pages, 2014. https://doi.org/10.1155/2014/240581

162. Jansen R. et al An integrative study of biological clocks in somatic and mental health eLife Journal 02/09/2021, accessed at eLife 2021;10:e59479 DOI: 10.7554/ eLife.59479

163. Hariprasad, V R et al. "Effects of yoga intervention on sleep and quality-of-life in elderly: A randomized controlled trial." *Indian journal of psychiatry* vol. 55,Suppl 3 (2013): S364-8. doi:10.4103/0019-5545.116310

164. Lawrence EM et al Happiness and Longevity in the United States, Soc Sci Med. 2015 Nov; 145: 115–119. Published online 2015 Sep 18. doi: 10.1016/j.socscimed.2015.09.020, Accessed from: https://www.ncbi.nlm.nih.gov/pmc/articles/PMC4724393/#:~:text=Academic%20interest%20in%20the%20study,over%20the%20past%20twenty%20years.&text=Extant%20research%20suggests%20that%20being,Chan%202011%3B%20Veenhoven%202008).

165. See notes about findings in Journal of Happiness Research at https://www.sciencedaily.com/releases/2008/08/080805075614.htm

Index